THE HYPERACTIVE CHILD,
ADOLESCENT, AND ADULT

THE HYPERACTIVE CHILD, ADOLESCENT, AND ADULT
Attention Deficit Disorder Through the Lifespan

Paul H. Wender

New York   Oxford
OXFORD UNIVERSITY PRESS
1987

Oxford University Press

Oxford   New York   Toronto
Delhi   Bombay   Calcutta   Madras   Karachi
Petaling Jaya   Singapore   Hong Kong   Tokyo
Nairobi   Dar es Salaam   Cape Town
Melbourne   Auckland

and associated companies in
Beirut   Berlin   Ibadan   Nicosia

Published by Oxford University Press, Inc.,
200 Madison Avenue, New York, New York 10016

Oxford is a registered trademark of Oxford University Press

Library of Congress Cataloging-in-Publication Data
Wender, Paul H., 1934-
   The hyperactive child, adolescent, and adult.
   Includes index.
   1. Attention deficit disorders. 2. Hyperactive child syndrome.
I. Title. [DNLM: 1. Attention Deficit Disorder with Hyperactivity. WS 340 W469h]
RJ496.A86W46   1987   616.85'89   86-12865
ISBN 0-19-504291-3
ISBN 0-19-504952-7 (pbk.)

This book was published in 1973 as *The Hyperactive Child* and
in 1978 as *The Hyperactive Child and the Learning Disabled Child*.

11
Printed in the United States of America
on acid-free paper.

Preface

In 1973 the first version of this book appeared, *The Hyperactive Child*, by Paul H. Wender. During several years of treating hyperactive children, my colleagues and I discovered that the parents of such children needed information about the nature, causes, and treatment of hyperactivity, and that no book was available with such data in a form suitable for the concerned layperson. *The Hyperactive Child* was written in response to this need, drawing on clinical and research experience as previously summarized in a book for physicians and other professionals working with children (P. H. Wender, *Minimal Brain Dysfunction in Children*. New York: Wiley, 1971).

In 1978 the second version of the book was published. The second edition contained new information about the medical and psychological management of hyperactivity, and also included a discussion of the learning disabilities that frequently—but not always—accompany hyperactivity.

This third version has been written for two reasons. One, it is a continuing update. Two, we have learned that problems associated with hyperactivity—which is now usually described as attention deficit disorder—are not necessarily outgrown and in many instances persist well into adult life. This third edition presents what we have learned about the symptoms, the diagnosis, and the treatment of hyperactivity in adults.

Although this edition does briefly describe the learning disabilities that often accompany hyperactivity, it devotes less attention to that topic than the previous edition did. The subject of learning disabilities (which frequently occur without hyperactivity) is a huge and controversial one, and the numerous experts in that area have an enormous variety of approaches to the different problems that may be encountered. Thus, I am limiting my coverage of that particular aspect of the functioning of some hyperactive children to a description that can alert parents to the possible need for special academic consultation.

As before, the book is dedicated to the hyperactive children and their families who have taught me so much about the disorder. It is dedicated also to those hyperactive adults who have educated me about their problems and have willingly participated in scientific experiments that taught all of us more about hyperactivity in adults. I continue to believe that better understanding will lead to better treatment of hyperactivity and learning disabilities, frequently misunderstood disorders of childhood, adolescence, and adulthood.

Salt Lake City   P.H.W
June 1986

Contents

THE HYPERACTIVE CHILD,
ADOLESCENT, AND ADULT

1

Introduction

There are probably five million "hyperactive" children in the United States. Although hyperactivity was described by physicians many years ago, its frequency has been recognized only recently. Exact figures are not available, but it seems likely that at least 3 to 10 percent of school-age children have hyperactivity problems, frequently accompanied by learning disabilities (often called dyslexia). Both hyperactivity and learning disabilities are much more common in boys, yet they can occur in girls as well.

Along with increasing awareness of the problem of hyperactivity, a better understanding of its causes and treatment has developed. The purpose of this book is to explain to parents the present understanding of this problem and the best techniques for its management. The book should of course be an aid, not a substitute for diagnosis and treatment by qualified physicians. It is designed to answer many of the most frequently asked questions and to describe some of the simple procedures that many parents have found helpful in dealing with their hyperactive children.

Although the behavioral problems that make up hyperactivity and the kinds of problems associated with learning disabilities often occur together in the same child, it is useful to view the disorders separately. First, not all hyperactive children have the problems in reading, spelling, and arithmetic that are seen in learning disabilities, and not all children with those kinds of learning disabilities have the behavioral difficulties of the hyperactive child. Second, the treatment of the behavior problems of hyperactivity and the treatment of the academic problems associated with learning disabilities are different. For the most part, therefore, I will discuss them separately.

A CHANGE OF NAMES

Hyperactivity has recently been rechristened by psychiatrists and given the new name of attention deficit disorder *with* hyperactivity. Attention deficit disorder (ADD) can also occur *without* hyperactivity. This renaming is useful. Previously, we had to talk about some hyperactive children who weren't hyperactive! Because these children had all the problems of attention deficit disorder except hyperactivity, they were diagnosed as nonhyperactive hyperactive children. Now they are simply ADD children without hyperactivity.

ADD children have been known by many different diagnostic names. Most of these emphasize either different aspects of the children's behavior or different theories of the origin of hyperactivity. Some synonyms for hyperactivity are maturational lag, hyperkinetic reaction, immaturity of the nervous system, and perceptual-motor problems. Two names for hyperactivity that are often misunderstood by parents are minimal brain dysfunction and minimal cerebral dysfunction. I hope that their meaning will become clearer in the course of my discussion. Finally, two fairly common names are usually incorrect: minimal brain damage and minimal brain injury. Although I will discuss the causes of hyperactivity later, I wish to emphasize now that most children with hyperactivity are *not* brain-damaged.

The terms *attention deficit disorder with hyperactivity* and *attention deficit disorder without hyperactivity* cover all these conditions. Although many scientific investigators use two abbreviations to distinguish between these two subvarieties of the disorder (ADDH and ADD), I will simply use the abbreviation ADD throughout the book to refer to either condition. In the overwhelming number of cases, hyperactivity is one of the symptoms of ADD.

A variety of problems that were formerly called learning disabilities also have a new name: specific developmental disorder (SDD). The most troublesome disability—reading problems—was often labeled dyslexia. The several different academic and nonacademic problems that are referred to by the term *specific developmental disorder* will be discussed later.

This book attempts to summarize what I have observed and learned in treating hundreds of ADD children over a period of more than fifteen years and what my colleagues and I have learned about ADD in adults during the past ten. In addition, it summarizes information obtained from the medical literature on the experiences and findings of other physicians.

In covering the subject of ADD, I will use the following words many times: few, some, frequently, many, most. In medicine and education one can rarely use such words as always, every, or never. The variety in people is stimulating in everyday life but complicating in medicine. Physicians would like to be able to use the words always or never, but seldom can. This may make approaching the subject more difficult, but it will present a more realistic picture.

2

The Characteristics of Children with Attention Deficit Disorder (ADD)

The task of describing the characteristics of children with attention deficit disorder (commonly described as hyperactive) is in some ways a difficult one. The attributes are not unusual, but many of the symptoms are present in all children to some degree at some particular time. Consequently, the parents reading this chapter are apt to conclude that all their children have attention deficit disorder (ADD). Before beginning, therefore, let me emphasize that the characteristics listed are not abnormal in themselves; they are only abnormal when they are excessive. What characterizes ADD children is the *intensity*, the *persistence*, and the *patterning* of these symptoms.

This chapter should not, of course, be used for diagnosis. Only a clinician who has evaluated many children can accurately decide if a given child has attention deficit disorder. Parents who try to make the diagnosis alone are like medical students who, after reading the symptoms of diseases in their texts, think they have contracted smallpox, leprosy, and cancer within the space of a few weeks. (Fortunately, they recover just as rapidly.) Parents who suspect that their restless, poorly coordinated, distractible, and demanding child may be hyperactive should seek the service of a competent specialist for diagnosis and a determination as to whether treatment is indeed indicated.

Finally, I wish to also emphasize that since the list of characteristics presented here is exhaustive, it does include some traits that are not necessarily present in all children with attention deficit disorder.

ATTENTION DIFFICULTIES AND DISTRACTIBILITY

One characteristic of the ADD child that is almost always present is easy distractibility or shortness of attention span. This difficulty is not as obvious as hyperactivity but is of greater practical importance. The ADD child does not have stick-to-itiveness.

Young children, in comparison to adults, are relatively lacking in the ability to concentrate and follow through on long and tedious tasks. The ADD child acts like a child younger than himself. He is the opposite of one who sits patiently in the corner painstakingly solving a puzzle and tolerating no interruptions. As a toddler and nursery school student, the ADD child rushes quickly from activity to activity, and then seems at a loss for things to do. In school his teacher reports: "You can't get him to pay attention for long. . . . He doesn't finish his work. . . . He doesn't follow instructions." (And how could an inattentive child do so if the teacher says, "Take your geography book, turn to page 43, think about the first three questions, and write the answers in your workbook"?)

At home his mother notices that "he doesn't listen for long . . . he doesn't mind . . . he doesn't remember." The parents must hover over the child to get him to do what they want. Told once to eat with his fork and not his hands, he complies, but a few seconds later he is eating with his hands again. He may begin his homework as requested but fail to complete it unless the parents nag him. The child may not necessarily disobey instructions, but in the middle of an assigned job he starts doing something else. Tasks begun are half done. His room is half restored to order; the lawn is half mowed. Sometimes, as discussed later, the child appears to remember but is reluctant to comply. Other times he appears to be distracted from the task at hand and forgets.

It is important to note that, like hyperactivity, distractibility need not be present at all times. Often when the child receives individual attention he can attend well for a while. The teacher may report that he "does well with one-to-one attention." A psychologist may note that the child can attend during testing. A pediatrician may observe that the child was not inattentive during the brief office examination. They are all correct, but what is important is not how the child can pay attention when an adult is exerting the maximum effort to get him to do so. Many ADD children can listen attentively for at least a little while. If the examiner, child psychiatrist, pediatrician, or psychologist does not realize the potential variability of such behavior, he or she may incorrectly come to the conclusion that the child is perfectly fine and that the parents and teacher are overreacting.

In *some* ADD children, the distractibility may be concealed by the ability to stick with a particular activity for an unusually long period of time. Usually it is an activity they choose themselves. Sometimes it is a socially useful one (e.g., reading), and sometimes it is not. The child may seem to "lock on" and be undetachable or unusually persistent. The activity may be repeated in a stereotyped and perseverative manner. Such paradoxical behavior in an ostensibly distractible child may confuse a parent, who will ask, "How can he be distractible when he plays with his rock collection for hours on end?" The highly unsatisfactory answer must be: "We do not know, but this is indeed the case."

IMPULSIVITY

A very frequently described characteristic of ADD children is "impulsivity" or "poor impulse control." Every young child wants what he wants when he wants it. He acts without reflection or consideration of the consequences. The ability to tolerate delays, to count to ten, to think before acting, tends to develop with age. Again, the ADD child behaves like a child several years younger than his chronological age.

He rapidly becomes upset when things or people fail to behave as he would have them behave. Toys get kicked (and sometimes broken), brothers and sisters and classmates are apt to get socked when they don't do what *they* should.

The ADD child acts on the spur of the moment. He rushes into the street, onto the ledge, up the tree. As a result he receives more than his share of cuts, bruises, abrasions, and trips to the doctor. He wears out clothes or destroys toys—not maliciously but unthinkingly. It seemed like fun to walk in the street in his Sunday best; he wondered what would happen if he pulled that knob on the toy.

Impulsivity is also shown in poor planning and judgment. It is difficult to specify how much planning and judgment one should expect of children, but, again, ADD children show less of these qualities than seems to be age appropriate. They are more likely than most children to run off in several directions at once. They are disorderly and disorganized. Their impulsivity combines with their distractibility to produce untidy rooms, sloppy dress (untucked shirts, unzipped zippers), unfinished assignments, careless reading and writing.

Another area that is a problem in some ADD children is bladder and bowel control, and it may be related to their impulsivity. When younger, some ADD children may wet or soil themselves slightly during the day. They seem to pay no attention to their "pressing needs" and overflow somewhat. Bed-wetting, which occurs in about 10 percent of all six-year-old boys, seems to be more common in ADD children. It may be that bed-wetting in some ADD children is related to unusually deep sleep, but this is not certain. The relationship between ADD and bed-wetting is important to recognize because "accidents" and bed-wetting are sometimes assumed to be a sign of anatomical abnormalities or deep psychological problems. Often, however, they are instead a manifestation of attention deficit disorder and respond to the general treatment prescribed for it.

Social impulsivity—antisocial behavior—is *sometimes* a problem in ADD children. At some time all children steal, all children lie, most children play with matches. As they grow older most chidren learn to inhibit these impulses. A few ADD children do not; they take, lie, or light matches whenever they want to. Now ADD itself does not explain *why* children wish to do these things. Children steal for a wide variety of reasons. Stealing may result from a simple desire to have or from a desire to have things that would buy affection; it may be an attempt to achieve status in a group; it may be a source of excitement; or it may be a means of retaliating, or obtaining attention or punishment. What is important is that if these motives occur in the ADD child, he is less able than other children to control himself. It should be obvious that treatment of such a child would require a twofold approach: dealing with the specific motivation and reducing the impulsivity (or increasing the ability for self-control).

HYPERACTIVITY

Not all ADD children are hyperactive (which is the reason the name of the disorder was changed). However, most ADD children are, and when hyperactivity is present it is very hard to miss. Many children with ADD have been excessively active since early infancy. Parents often report that the child was "different" from the beginning of his life. Frequently, such infants are restless and have feeding problems and colic (intermittent and unexplained crying). They also often have sleeping problems of various sorts: some children fall asleep late and with difficulty, awaken frequently, and arise early; others fall asleep profoundly and are hard to arouse.

As these infants become toddlers, many of them are bundles of energy. The parents frequently report that after an active and restless infancy, the child stood and walked at an early age, and then, like an infant King Kong, burst the bars of his crib and marched forth to destroy the house. He was always on the go, always into everything, always touching (and hence, usually by mistake, breaking) every object in sight. When unwatched for a moment he somehow got to the top of the refrigerator or appeared in the middle of the street. In a twinkling, pots and pans were whisked from cupboards, ashtrays knocked off tables, and lamps overturned. The mother usually felt—and with good cause—that to take her eyes off him for one moment was to invite disaster: the moment her back was turned, something was broken or the toddler's life was in danger. And she was right. ADD children have more than their share of accidents and are much more likely than non-ADD children to be seen in emergency rooms.

As the ADD child grows older the description changes: he is incessantly in motion, driven like a motor, constantly fidgeting, drumming his fingers, shuffling his feet. He does not stay at any activity long. He pulls all his toys off the shelf, plays with each for a moment and discards it. He cannot color for long. He cannot be read to without quickly losing interest. Of course he is unable to keep from squirming at the dinner table; he may not even be able to sit still in front of the TV set. In the car he drives the other passengers wild. He opens and closes ashtrays, plays with the windows, tugs others' seat belts, and kicks the passengers in the front seat. At school his teacher relates that the child is fidgety, disruptive, unable to sit still in his seat; that he gets up and walks around the classroom, talks out, clowns; and that he jostles, bothers, and annoys his fellow pupils. Sometimes the ADD child is as overtalkative as he is overactive, talking as ceaselessly as he moves.

It is important to emphasize that what is different about the ADD child is not his level of activity while at play. All children make all adults look like sloths. The ADD child cannot be distinguished on the playground. His top speed is not greater than that of other children. What is so different about the ADD child is that when he is requested to turn off his motor, he cannot do so for very long. Unlike other children, he cannot inhibit his activity in the home or the classroom. However, the ADD child need not *always be* moving. Sometimes he can sit relatively still. For whatever reason, this is most apt to occur when he is getting individual attention from an adult. That is worth remembering because sometimes people who examine the child are misled when he sits more or less still for 10 to 15 minutes. They usually discover their error when they try to increase that time to an hour or so.

To repeat, an important point about ADD is that *not all ADD children are hyperactive*. There are ADD children who have many of the problems I'm discussing but are not overactive at all, and there are even a few who are less than normally active. These ADD children are more likely to be overlooked than those with hyperactive ADD. This is particularly likely if they have learned to keep quiet as a way of avoiding embarrassment. *All the other problems can exist without hyperactivity itself.*

The second point is that clear-cut hyperactivity may be the first symptom to disappear as the child grows older. (However, it may simply remain in a less obvious form. The ADD adolescent or adult may continually fidget or tap a foot and may describe himself as restless, unable to sit still for long, and prefer energetic to quiet activities.) Often the other problems persist. Therefore, even though a child was once overactive but no longer is does not mean that all problems are resolved. Many other problems may continue to require treatment even though the hyperactivity itself is gone.

ATTENTION-DEMANDING BEHAVIOR

In order to develop normally, all children require adult interest, involvement, and attention. As they grow older, they require less but still need the awareness and interest of those whom they love and respect.

The ADD child demands attention but this in itself is not what makes him different. He is different and difficult because of his insatiability. Like a younger child he wants to be always on center stage. He may whine, badger, tease, and annoy without stop. The manifestations change with age. As a toddler he may repeat annoying and prohibited activities; as an older child he may attempt to monopolize the dinner-table conversation, clown in the classroom, and show off with his friends at the risk of his neck and to the distress of law enforcement agencies.

These aspects of his behavior may be concealed by the fact that he sometimes does not manifest certain kinds of affectionate behavior. Many, although far from all, ADD children have been undemonstrative. In infancy they were noncuddlers. They did not go to sleep on laps but wiggled off to go about their own business. They were not upset when their mothers left them with baby-sitters or at nursery school.

Nonetheless, the same children sometimes figuratively managed to stand at arm's length and prod their parents with a pole.

The demand for attention can be distressing, confusing, and irritating to parents. Since the child demands so much they feel they have not given him what he needs. Since they cannot understand how to satisfy him, they feel deficient. Finally, because the child may cling and poke simultaneously and endlessly, they feel angry.

SCHOOL DIFFICULTIES

In discussing the school difficulties that sometimes afflict ADD children, it is important to emphasize that ADD does *not* affect intelligence as ordinarily defined and measured by intelligence tests. The proportions of the bright, normal, and slow are the same among ADD children as among children who do not have ADD. Attention deficit disorder is not in any way related to mental retardation.

However, *some* ADD children, not all, do have certain problems in intellectual development and in perception. Some may have an "unevenness" of intellectual development. Intelligence tests measure abilities and skills in a number of separate areas, such as vocabulary, arithmetic, understanding, memory, and certain forms of problem solving. Usually a child's performance is pretty much the same in each of these separate areas. If a child's vocabulary is normal for his age, his memory and problem solving are usually age-normal as well. ADD children seem more likely to have uneven development. Thus, an ADD child's intelligence, which averages his ability in all these areas, may be average but he may be advanced in some and behind in others. This can produce difficulties in school placement and adjustment. A hyperactive child in the third grade may be able to do fifth-grade mathematics but only second-grade reading. If the school does not make allowances for these inconsistent abilities, the problems of such a child will be accentuated. He cannot be moved to a regular fifth or second grade, for he will be too slow for one and too fast for the other.

Unless the school can arrange a program to take his abilities into account, he will not fit into *any* class.

Such children *sometimes* require special learning techniques and tutoring. The area of perception in which *some* ADD children have problems is a difficult one to define. It is more complex than simple seeing or hearing. It includes the abilities to distinguish between similar sights or sounds and the ability to put together sensations in a meaningful way.

For example, one perceptual task that sometimes can give an ADD child trouble is the problem of distinguishing between right and left. Young children have difficulty learning the difference between right and left and gradually learn to tell directions apart by the age of five or six. Young children confuse their right and left hands and feet and are apt to put their gloves on the wrong hands and their shoes on the wrong feet. Some ADD children appear to be slow in learning the right-left concept (and a *very* few may also have problems in distinguishing between up and down). Problems in distinguishing between right and left seem associated with problems in reading.

"Perceptual" difficulties of this kind, and related difficulties, in children of normal intelligence, are called specific developmental disorders (SDD). It is important to remember that many children with ADD do not have SDD, and that many children with SDD do not have ADD. Correct diagnosis is essential in planning rational medical, psychological, and educational treatment.

As I indicated in the Introduction, SDD is the new phrase that replaces learning disability. The two most common SDDs are in reading (and spelling) and arithmetic. The formal diagnostic names are developmental reading disorder and developmental arithmetic disorder.

The feature that all SDDs have in common is that children (and adults) with them have problems performing in these academic areas even though they have no serious psychiatric illness, possess adequate intelligence, and receive adequate teaching. SDDs are called developmental problems because it is believed that they are the result of a slow maturational process in specific areas. We do not use the term developmental reading disorder for children who are intellectually slow in many areas, including reading. Such children are equally and predictably slow in a wider range of areas, so that one would expect them to have difficulty in reading. Individuals with SDDs have a discrepancy between their intelligence and their performance in reading and/or spelling and/or arithmetic. For example, consider a ten-year-old third grader with average intelligence. He or she should be reading at a ten-year-old level. If he is only reading as well as an average eight year old, he is two years behind and may be diagnosed as having a developmental disorder in reading.

Two questions about SDDs are usually asked by parents. The first is "How can a child get a normal score on an intelligence test and have trouble with reading?" The answer is that the kind of intelligence tests that are used to diagnose suspected SDD do not involve reading. The psychologist *asks* questions of the child, and the test is designed to measure such things as knowledge, abstraction, reasoning, memory, problem solving, observational ability, and quickness. We do not know enough about the brain and mind to know why someone can be very smart and yet be unable to read well or unable to add up a column of numbers, but we do know that many such people exist. I have seen children and adults with marked SDDs who read painfully slowly or who cannot add figures in their checkbook (or scientific experiments!) but who play a brilliant game of chess, are sophisticated inventors, or are at home in advanced mathematics. Such uneven development has important practical consequences, of course, both for education and for the psychological well-being of the person with an SDD.

The second question usually asked is "How far behind does someone have to be to be diagnosed as having an SDD?" There is no scientific reason for selecting a particular number, but generally school systems say 24 months or two years. Thus, SDDs are often not definitely diagnosed until the third grade. Then, if a child is two years behind, he can be identified as reading like a normal first grader. However, although it is difficult to diagnose SDDs before the third grade, parents and teachers are often correct in suspecting such problems when the first- or second-grade child is lagging far behind the other children in learning to read.

In developmental reading disorder one sees the following: difficulties in reading out loud, together with adding, omitting, and changing words. In spelling to dictation there are frequent errors. Letters may be reversed ("b" confused with "d") or transposed. Handwriting is often horrendous—illegible and unplanned, wandering all over the page. Children with an SDD in arithmetic often reverse figures in columns and show difficulties with word problems (if apples are 3¢ each and I buy eight and give you a quarter, how much do you owe me?). In addition to these relatively specific problems, children with SDDs often have various other problems, such as the previously mentioned difficulty in telling right from left. Some have trouble with spatial relations—the person cannot follow directions to find his way around a strange place or city. Sometimes the child has difficulty in learning sequences (such as the days of the week or the months of the year) or in telling time (before the invention of the digital watch!). For others learning and retaining the multiplication table presents special problems.

Some experts who have studied SDD think that problems in reading can usefully be thought of as falling into different categories. One well-known investigator, Elena Boder, has suggested a tentative two-part classification that many workers in the field find helpful. Boder divides SDD children into two overlapping groups: auditory-language dyslexics (A-dyslexics) and visual-spatial dyslexics (V-dyslexics). The A-dyslexic has a good visual memory but has difficulty with phonetics— that is, he has trouble relating isolated sounds and the small groups of letters on the printed page that refer to syllables. If he knows a word, he knows it as a whole. He will be able to read and spell words that he has previously mastered. But because he has not grasped phonetics he has trouble in reading and spelling unfamiliar words.

The V-dyslexic understands phonetics. He can sound out new words, and if they are phonetic he can often do so correctly. Similarly, he will spell unfamiliar words phonetically. However, he has a higher than normal number of letter and word reversals and omissions.

Boder believes that A-dyslexia is four to five times as common as V-dyslexia, although many children have a mixture of both problems.

She believes that other problems are specifically associated with A- and V-dyslexia. For example, she finds that A-dyslexics tend to do better in problem solving than in verbal parts of intelligence tests, and that V-dyslexia is sometimes accompanied by difficulty in distinguishing between right and left and by poor handwriting.

I cannot emphasize too much that it is possible to have these problems and still be intelligent. Many fine athletes, musicians, and mechanics have SDD. There are numerous ways in which children and adults with SDDs can compensate for their deficiencies. Eminent people known for high achievement have had SDDs—for example, Thomas Edison and Harvey Cushing (the father of neurosurgery) had severe dyslexia. Academic skills represent only one part of the vast range of human skills and they have become more important only recently, as literacy has become widespread.

It is useful to compare people with SDDs with tone-deaf people. Tone-deaf people generally have normal hearing and normal intelligence but have difficulty in reproducing musical pitch accurately. They have trouble, for example, singing in tune or playing the violin. Everyone understands that one can be very intelligent and yet be unable to carry a tune. If singing were important and reading were not—as in some primitive tribes—tone deaf people would be handicapped as if they had an SDD. In hunting societies, speed and coordination would be the most important skills; dyslexia (and tone deafness) would be irrelevant. Thus dyslexia is a culture-dependent disorder.

Nevertheless, we must not underestimate the importance of these SDDs, which we think are physically produced. Having trouble in reading or arithmetic not only makes progress difficult in the academic and business worlds but also leads to typical psychological problems. I will return to these problems in later chapters.

Remember that many ADD children have none of these perceptual problems. Nevertheless, most ADD children have considerable difficulty in learning at school. "Underachievement" is almost a hallmark of the ADD child. Teachers and guidance counselors will, of course, recognize that the child has problems, and sometimes the school is the first place that the child's problems are clearly recognized. However, school personnel sometimes underestimate the problems related to ADD and may attribute the child's difficulties to emotional problems, psychological maladjustment, or problems in the home.

If the ADD child does *not* have specific perceptual problems, there are several possible explanations for his poor school performance. All his learning problems may stem from the attention difficulties and emotional overreactivity that have already been discussed. An eight-year-old with ADD, despite normal intelligence, may be reacting to the school in the same fashion as a normal four or five year old. Intelligence is not enough. A child must have the ability to concentrate for a reasonable period of time; he must hear at least *some* of what is said if he is to learn. He must have a reasonable amount of stick-to-itiveness and patience to tolerate difficult tasks; if he gives up immediately, learning will obviously be impaired. And, as has been mentioned several times, the ADD child is both inattentive and readily frustrated. The learning problems are further complicated because they tend to move in vicious circles; they often snowball. His poor performance is apt to cause the teacher to say, either in so many words or indirectly: "Why can't you use your brains? . . . Why don't you finish your work? . . . Do your work. . . . You could if you wanted to." Thus poor performance leads to criticism, which in turn leads to the child's having a poor opinion of himself. Both are likely to decrease his motivation to do well. If he can't do well when he is trying to the best of his ability, he tends to give up. The result is a performance that grows steadily worse. If a child is a bit slow in the first few grades, he remains at a disadvantage even if most of the ADD disappears and his learning ability catches up. Since he is now behind academically, school is harder and more frustrating.

Finally, much of any school experience is boring, tedious, repetitious. Many parents who visit an elementary school for the first time in ten or twenty years are impressed with its tedium and wonder how they were able to pay attention when they were children. This is not to say that making school into a consistently interesting experience would eliminate the ADD child's difficulties. Probably it would not. I only mean to point out that the social structure in most schools makes the ADD child's problems greater.

DIFFICULTIES IN COORDINATION

Approximately half of ADD children show various difficulties in coordination. Some ADD children have limited "fine-motor control": they have trouble coloring, cutting with scissors, tying shoelaces, and buttoning. Handwriting is often terrible and the ADD child perceives writing as a chore. The combination of poor coordination and failure to plan can lead to an illegible written page, with words overrunning lines, the sides of the page, and each other. Others may have some mild difficulty with balance—for example, in learning to ride a bicycle. Still other ADD children may have poor hand-eye coordination: these children will be awkward in throwing and catching a ball or in playing baseball or tennis. Not all ADD children have such problems. Many are well coordinated and some are excellent athletes. When coordination problems are present they usually cause more difficulties for boys than for girls because for boys athletic ability is an important source of acceptance by others. However, even the children with coordination handicaps may have no problems in activities requiring large muscle groups and may run or swim without difficulty.

RESISTANT AND DOMINEERING SOCIAL BEHAVIOR

Most hyperactive children manifest interpersonal behavior that has several distinct characteristics: (1) a considerable resistance to social demands, a resistance to "dos" and "don'ts," to "shoulds" and "shouldn'ts" (this is a frequent cause of difficulty with parents and teachers); (2) increased independence; (3) domineering behavior with other children.

Probably the single most disturbing feature of ADD children's behavior, and the one most frequently responsible for their referral for treatment, is the difficulty many of these children have in complying with requests and prohibitions of parents and teachers. Some ADD children may appear almost impossible to discipline. In some respects they seem to remain two years old. Parents describe them as "obstinate

. . . stubborn . . . negativistic . . . bossy . . . disobedient . . . sassy . . . not caring." All the techniques of discipline seem unsuccessful: rewards, removal of privileges, physical punishment. "He wants his own way. . . . He never seems to hear. . . . He never learns by his own mistakes. . . . You can't reach him. . . . Punishment just rolls off his back. . . . He's almost immune to anything we do." ADD children differ, however, in the ways they manifest resistance. Some seem to forget what they are told, whereas others seem to oppose actively what is requested of them. I will discuss the meaning of this when I discuss the causes of the disorder.

With regard to independence, the ADD child is often excessively independent but in a few instances is excessively dependent. The independence may be noticed at an early age. The ADD child is the sort of child apt to wander ten blocks away from home when he is two years old. When he is brought home to his terrified and angry parents, he is smiling and excited. He does not seem to get upset by the separation. He is *not* the sort of child who is likely to be upset the first few days of nursery school or kindergarten or when left with his grandparents. The few ADD children at the other extreme, those who are excessively dependent, tend to be immature, babyish, and clinging. They are the children most likely to show the incessant attention-demanding behavior that I have described.

The ADD child's relationships with his brothers, sisters, and school-mates are likely to follow a clearly recognizable pattern. When he is younger he tends to be a tease. He becomes quite expert at getting others' goats, annoying, and bothering. As he grows older, he shows a very marked tendency to be bossy. Note how this contrasts with his refusal to be bossed by adults. When he plays with other children he strives to be the leader. He wants to decide what games will be played. He wants to decide what the rules are, and if the game is not played the way he likes he may quit: he wants to play it his way or not at all. Needless to say, this does not win friends and influence people (at least favorably). Other children tend to avoid him, and after a while the ADD child is likely to be without friends. This lack of friendship is much different from what one sees in a shy, withdrawn child. The

ADD child is usually aggressive socially and *initiates* friendship successfully, but his style drives other children away. He will tell his parents that he is talked about, rejected, and perhaps even bullied. These reports are not excuses and they are not inaccurate. They are correct reports of what his own behavior compels other children to do. He "makes friends easily but can't keep them." As a result, the ADD child often plays with younger children, and for the same reason the ADD boy sometimes plays with girls. However, the ADD child is not necessarily physically aggressive. He is not sadistic and does not enjoy hurting others. He *does* tend to have more than his share of fights, but this is because of his impulsivity and because brothers and sisters and schoolmates are usually not enthusiastic about being pushed around and told what to do.

EMOTIONAL DIFFICULTIES

Most ADD children show certain forms of emotional problems. The word emotional is one of those vague terms used by everyone in a variety of ways whose meaning is not clear. Let me emphasize first that calling these problems emotional does *not* imply that they are psychologically caused. Indeed, most of them are probably not psychologically caused.

ADD children tend to have mood swings and cycles, so that their behavior tends to be unpredictable. Parents report: "He's happy one minute, impossible to get along with the next. . . . He has his good days and bad days, and it's hard to understand why." The last statement is important. All of us have our good and bad days, and often we can link our moods to our experiences. In the case of the ADD child, it is usually more difficult to find out why he was bad yesterday and good today.

Many ADD children are unusually underreactive and overreactive. They are sometimes insensitive to pain. They seem unaffected by and rarely react to the frequent bumps, falls, and scrapes that are the lot of younger children. (This is sometimes obscured by increased attention-seeking. When their parents are looking they may tend to squeeze out every last drop of sympathy obtainable.) They are often relatively fearless. A combination of this fearlessness, a craving for attention, impulsivity, and a tendency not to "plan ahead" is apt to land them in socially unapproved situations: when young, at the tops of trees; when older, impressing their adolescent peers with taboo behavior and inviting the interest of the local police. Fortunately, such fearlessness is *not* seen in all ADD children.

The overreactivity of ADD children sometimes manifests itself in excessive excitement during pleasant activities. Most young children will be excited at the circus, but ADD children tend to become very overexcited in such circumstances. They may even lose control of themselves in less stimulating situations, for example, during a visit to a supermarket.

The overreactivity can also be seen in excessive irritability or anger during frustrating activities. Of course, most children (and adults) do not tolerate frustration or disappointment very well. But the ADD child has a much lower tolerance for frustration and a more violent reaction to it. When things do not go his way he is subject to temper tantrums, angry outbursts, or sullen spells. Most young children become irritable and babyish when tired or hungry. An eight-year-old ADD child may react to fatigue or hunger in the same way that a normal four year old does.

Although many parents describe their ADD children as "angry," what they usually seem to be referring to is irritability and hot temper rather than aggressiveness or hostility, that is, hyperreactivity to comparative minor situations: "He's got a low boiling point . . . a short fuse. . . . When he's angry he loses control." Many ADD children are described as being good-natured except during such outbursts.

One other characteristic seen in some ADD children that is frequently disturbing to parents might be called "unsatisfiability." "He never gets a kick out of anything, at least not for long. . . . He can't be bothered to do much, nothing really seems to give him pleasure. . . . You can never satisfy him." This characteristic is sometimes produced by spoiling (in adults as well as children), but many ADD children behave this way without ever having been spoiled. Their mothers may have noticed that they were not satisfiable from early infancy.

Finally, one "emotional" characteristic of most ADD children is also found in many children with other difficulties: low self-esteem. They have little self-confidence: "He doesn't think much of himself. . . . He thinks he's bad. . . . He thinks he's different." The cause and the treatment of such low self-esteem will be discussed at greater length later.

IMMATURITY

Immaturity is neither a very scientific nor a very specific word, but it often does accurately describe the behavior of ADD children. Their lack of social, athletic, and academic skills, their inability to remember—and act on—"dos and don'ts," are certainly characteristic of younger children. The inability to tolerate frustration (often resulting in tantrums) and the lack of stick-to-itiveness, are normal in younger children. Finally, some ADD children have another trait associated with immaturity: rigidity, the inability to tolerate change (such children will be upset if their routine is changed, if the furniture in their room is rearranged, etc.). From a practical standpoint, it is often helpful for parents to rememer that emotionally, not intellectually, their ADD child may behave very much like a child four or five years younger than he is. Remembering this often makes it easier for parents to handle their child; many parents do not know how to act toward a nine year old with problems but do know how to deal with a normal four or five year old. If the parents can remember that their ADD nine year old is in some respects acting like a normal five year old, they may find it easier to understand and help him.

CHANGING PROBLEMS WITH AGE

A salient aspect of the ADD child's problems is that they tend to change as he grows older. The behavioral problems that are conspicuous in a toddler are very different from those in an adolescent.

There are several reasons for this. First, there seem to be changes associated with maturation; for example, the symptoms themselves tend to diminish with age (just as bed-wetting disappears with age). Second, some changes occur as a result of learning: the ADD child is more hostile after his tenth year of rejection by schoolmates than he is after only one or two years of such treatment. Third, recognition of "problems" depends on one's understanding of the behavior considered normal for particular age groups: fidgety behavior is expected and tolerated in nursery school children but not in second graders; reading difficulty is expected in all first graders but is a problem in fourth grade.

What is the usual sequence of difficulties? In infancy the ADD child's most conspicuous problems are in physiologic function: he is likely to be irritable, to have colic, and to have sleep disturbances. During the toddler stage his ability to do things increases immensely, and many of them are troublesome things. The most disturbing traits are his continual "getting into" things and his inability to listen, that is, to respond to parental discipline.

As he reaches preschool age, his problems with attention and social adjustment claim the limelight. His short attention span, low frustration tolerance, and temper tantrums make sustained play and nursery school participation difficult. Problems with his schoolmates soon appear: teasing, domination, and other annoying behaviors. These qualities endear him neither to his teacher nor to his fellows, and in a few instances result in his beginning his academic career as a kindergarten dropout.

When he starts the first grade, his restlessness attracts attention: his teacher complains that he cannot sit still, that he gets up and walks around, whistles, and shuffles. Academic problems, though often present, tend to be ignored. First graders are not expected to read immediately. Bed-wetting may now appear. Although he may have always been a bed-wetter, bed-wetting is defined as a problem only when the child reaches an age when it is expected to disappear (usually about six), or when he stays overnight at camp or with friends. At about the third grade, when the child is nine or ten, academic and antisocial problems attract the most attention. Until that time slowness in school

℞Dermovate®

**Cream, Ointment and
Dermovate Scalp Application**

*For acute conditions and
flare-ups.*

℞Eumovate®

Cream and Ointment

*For maintenance and
chronic conditions.*

Glaxo Laboratories

can be attributed to immaturity or academic unreadiness. But in the third grade the diagnosis is changed to learning problems or learning disability. Reading difficulty causes the greatest concern, but the child may also have trouble with arithmetic and be criticized for messy writing. Outside of school, antisocial behavior is likely to be the cause of considerable concern. Both the duration and intensity of these problems are highly variable.

If the problems persist into early adolescence, the antisocial problems become the focus of attention. If academic problems persist, they may now be taken for granted. This is not to say that the same child who has a reading problem predictably develops social problems. Rather, if the child has both reading and social problems, the social problems attract the greatest concern at this time.

I wish to emphasize very strongly that the age patterns I have described do not apply to all ADD children. Some children manifest difficulties in all developmental stages, some in only a few. At any one stage, the difficulties vary from child to child: some will have academic problems, some will have coordination problems, some will have learning problems, some will have social problems, some will have different combinations of these problems, and an unfortunate few will have all of them.

Finally, many ADD children tend to outgrow not only their hyperactivity but also a large proportion of the associated other difficulties. Any given ADD child may follow the developmental sequence listed and then may no longer manifest ADD characteristics at a later stage, say, as a preadolescent. In fact, it is not uncommon for the problems to diminish or become easily manageable at or around the time of puberty.

The combination of problems that are seen among ADD children constitutes what is called a syndrome in medical terminology. A syndrome is a group of difficulties that *tend* to clump, cluster, or move together. It is characteristic of medical syndromes for a given individual not to have all the problems associated with the syndrome. It is also important to note that the child who does not have some of the problems listed at any given stage in his development is very unlikely to develop them at a later stage. The child who does not have coordination problems when he is young will not get them when he is older. The child who does not have reading problems when he is seven or eight will not have them as a teen-ager. To the parents burdened with those difficulties that their ADD child does have, this optimistic aspect of his development may be of some comfort. It is not to be minimized, for it has been observed by physicians who have treated these children and worked with their families over periods of years.

For those ADD children who do continue to have problems related to the disorder in adolescence and adulthood, research suggests that a combination of the various treatments available for ADD can lead to a better prognosis. I will describe in greater detail what is known about ADD in adolescents and adults in later chapters.

3

The Causes of Attention Deficit Disorder

In virtually all instances, attention deficit disorder is the result of an inborn temperamental difference in the child. How the child is treated and raised can affect the severity of his problem but it cannot cause the problem. Certain types of raising may make the problem worse, certain types may make the problem better. No forms of raising can produce ADD problems in a child who is not temperamentally predisposed to them.

Since child-rearing techniques can to some degree affect the seriousness of the ADD child's problem, changes in these techniques are usually helpful. They will be discussed in the chapter on treatment. Even though such psychological approaches can be helpful in the management of the ADD child, this does not affect the explanation of the origin of the syndrome—the basic source of the difficulties seems to be inborn.

CAUSES OF THE TEMPERAMENTAL PROBLEMS

Knowledge about the origin of attention deficit disorder is very incomplete, but evidence from various scientific areas is beginning to indicate that the two major causes of ADD seem to be: (1) an exaggeration or an excess of traits that normally vary from person to person; (2) a genetically determined disorder. It is very important to emphasize first, as I mentioned earlier, that *most ADD children are not brain damaged*. ADD children are sometimes referred to as brain damaged because ADD was first described in children who had suffered injuries to the brain. The term brain damaged not only is inaccurate but also is understandably upsetting to parents, who interpret it to mean that something is irreversibly the matter with the child's brain. In the few instances in which brain damage is the cause, parents should be less pessimistic than they usually are. This will be discussed in the chapter on the development of the ADD child.

If brain damage is not the cause, what is? Recent scientific evidence supports what everyone's grandmother knew: there are inborn temperamental differences among children. Studies of the growth of children from infancy to preadolescence reveal that children differ from their earliest days and that some of these differences tend to be associated with behavioral problems as the child grows up. For example, the difficulties that the ADD child is likely to have in infancy (colic, feeding problems, sleeping problems) are probably the result of inborn temperamental differences. What causes these differences? Child psychiatrists are not certain. A very good possibility is that they are caused by chemical differences in the brain. The brain is an extraordinarily complex interconnection of nerve cells. In some ways it is analogous to a telephone network, but with one major difference. In the telephone network the connections are *electrical*: electricity passes from one wire to another by physical contact. In the brain, however, the connections are *chemical*. One nerve cell releases a small amount of certain chemicals, which are picked up by a second cell, causing it to "fire." These chemicals are called neurotransmitters. If there is too little of a particular neurotransmitter, the second cell will not fire because not enough of the neurotransmitter has been released by the first cell. Although the nerve cells themselves are intact, it is as if the connection were broken. There are different neurotransmitters in different portions of the brain. If the amount of one neurotransmitter is insufficient, the portion of the brain that it operates will not function correctly. ADD children are probably deficient in some neurotransmitters. (In many ADD children the quantity of these transmitters probably increases with age. This would seem to be the likely reason that children improve as they grow older. This, too, will be discussed in the next chapter.)

The causes of these presumed chemical differences are, again, unknown but there are two general possibilities: (1) anomalies in the development of the baby *before* the time of birth; (2) genetic differences. Little is known about prenatal influences but there is some possibility that small birth size—and therefore prematurity—may sometimes lead to ADD symptoms. Similarly, other variations in the mother's biological processes during pregnancy might result in fetal maldevelopment. With regard to genetic origins, it has long been observed that ADD and reading problems sometimes run in families (and usually among the males when they do). It has also been learned that such traits as hair color, eye color, certain forms of mental deficiency, etc., are related to the production of particular chemicals of the body, and that the amounts and types of these chemicals are determined by the genes—the transmitters of inherited characteristics. Certain genes may also control the amounts of neurotransmitters and some genes result in too little production of the neurotransmitters. Neurochemists have some possible leads about which neurotransmitters may be insufficient in ADD children. These chemicals are located in that portion of the brain that includes among its functions the regulation of attention. An excess of these neurotransmitters might produce an increased ability to focus attention and to inhibit behavior, to control oneself. A deficiency in these neurotransmitters—which is probably the condition present in ADD children—would produce an underactivity of that portion of the brain, resulting in attention difficulties and some lack of self-control. This portion of the brain probably also acts to modulate the mood and increase appropriate reactions to things going on outside the child. Therefore, deficiency in neurotransmitters in this area would result in a decreased ability to focus attention; a decreased ability to check one's behavior—to apply brakes; a decreased sensitivity to others' reactions—to dos and don'ts, and approval or disapproval; and a decreased ability to modulate mood, that is, an increased tendency toward sudden and dramatic mood changes.

It is a common observation that particular kinds of temperament tend to run in families. In some families the children are high strung (like fox terriers or cocker spaniels), whereas in others the children are more placid. Any temperamental characteristic is not an all-or-none trait. It is like height. There are all degrees of tallness, from the very short to the very tall. Most people who are very short or very tall do not suffer from a disease, although it may be very inconvenient to be 4'6" or 7'2". Similarly, most degrees of high-strungness do not cause problems unless they are excessive. All the traits of ADD children that I have discussed occur in all children. At times, all children have short attention spans, are restless, and intolerant of not getting what they want. ADD children have these characteristics to a marked degree. They are often, in a sense, extremes of the normal, as are very short or very tall people. Their characteristics are too much and too little of certain normal traits.

In families in which ADD occurs on a temperamental basis, parents will frequently tell us that they had similar problems themselves when they were the age of their ADD son or daughter. Being aware of this similarity can be useful or harmful, depending on the circumstances. It can be an advantage when the parents remember the problems they faced and the techniques that were most helpful in dealing with them. This may provide useful insight for helping the child. The awareness can be harmful when the parents play down the difficulties from ADD. If the parents are unwilling to acknowledge that ADD caused them difficulty (or still does), they may minimize the problems it is causing the child. If this happens, the parents may neglect serious problems that require recognition in order to be alleviated.

As scientists have studied ADD children, they have begun to examine the psychological problems encountered among close relatives, particularly siblings and parents. They have observed two important things. First, the siblings of ADD children are more likely to have ADD problems than are the siblings of children without ADD. Second, as indicated above, the fathers and other close male relatives of ADD children report that they had such problems themselves as children (and, as we will see later, many probably have them as adults).

The psychiatrists who made these observations did not know at first whether the disorder was really hereditary or not. Perhaps parents who were psychologically disturbed brought up psychologically disturbed children. This would not be genetic but would be a form of psychological heredity. Not everything that runs in families is genetic. And how strongly something runs in a family doesn't tell us if it is transmitted genetically or through learning. All of the offspring of Chinese-speaking parents speak Chinese—this is 100 percent learned. A fairly small fraction of the children of a red-headed parent have red hair—and having red hair is a trait that is hereditarily transmitted. The problem is one of separating nature and nurture.

Investigators have tackled this problem in an ingenious way. They have studied adopted ADD children, or ADD children raised by foster parents, which permits them to separate the influence of genetic factors from the influence of family upbringing. Such studies indicate, for example, that (1) full siblings of ADD children are twice as likely as half siblings to have ADD themselves; (2) many cases of special developmental disorder (learning disabilities) are genetic in origin (particularly among males); (3) ADD *may* sometimes be associated with other disorders that seem strongly affected by genetic factors (alcoholism is one possibility).

Although these genetic findings suggest that certain types of parents are more likely to have ADD children, the studies do not indicate that such parents will inevitably have ADD children.

There are a number of other possible causes of ADD physicians are only now becoming aware of. The first is lead poisoning. It has been known for a long time that people who absorb too much lead develop both psychological and neurological (damage to nerves) problems. In fact, it was known thirty years ago that some children who ate lead (usually in the form of lead paint on walls, windowsills, or cribs) developed hyperactivity. What has recently been discovered is that lead poisoning may develop in children who never consumed lead. Studies in big cities have suggested that some children who are diagnosed as hyperactive have mild, chronic lead poisoning. The reason for this is unknown. One very unpleasant possibility is that merely living in heavily trafficked areas and breathing air containing automobile fumes may be sufficient to develop lead poisoning. As everyone undoubtedly realizes, a chemical compound containing lead has long been used in gasoline to improve the performance of cars. When the gasoline is burned, the lead is heated, becomes a gas, and passes into the air. In large cities, it may be sufficient merely to breathe the air to take in too much lead. Whether there is enough lead in the air in small-and medium-sized towns to allow for the same possibility is as yet unknown.

Another possible cause of ADD was proposed by a West Coast allergist (a physician specializing in the diagnosis and treatment of allergies, including asthma, hay fever, and allergic reactions to foods), who claimed that hyperactivity may be caused by the food children eat.

These claims received serious attention from a number of scientific investigators, who conducted controlled experiments on the effect of food additives. In controlled experiments, the investigator makes allowances for people's expectation about a treatment. If people believe they are receiving a helpful treatment but actually are not, they will often respond satisfactorily, even though their difficulties are entirely physical and not mental. An example is that of soldiers who received "million dollar wounds"—injuries that resulted in discharge from the Army but not permanent impairment: one-third of these soldiers who received a dummy injection (a placebo) rather than morphine felt no pain. Thus, if ADD children participate in an experiment that they believe might help them, conceivably they might function better on the basis of that belief alone.

There are two other reasons ADD children receiving a special diet might function better or appear to function better. First, their parents want to see a change. Because they are so eager to see improvement in their child, they may judge his behavior inaccurately. Since the researcher depends on the parent to describe the child's behavior at home, he may come to the wrong conclusion about the child's possible improvement. Second, an ADD child placed on a special diet might really do better because he becomes the center of much more attention. A diet without food additives usually requires a great deal of home preparation of foods. To the extent that increased attention can (perhaps temporarily) improve a child's behavior, an ADD child will actually do better under these circumstances.

As a control for such problems, experimenters used an innovative approach. They arranged with families of ADD children to remove all the food from the house. Each week the head of the house ordered the food the family would need for that week and the experimenters supplied all of it. With the permission of participating families, the experimenters sometimes included additives in the food and sometimes did not, but did not inform the families about those changes in the food. The investigators then examined the children's behavior both at home and in school. What they found is that the presence of food additives did not affect children to any appreciable degree. Their problems persisted when food additives were deleted, and their problems did not become worse when food additives were reinserted.

Another factor sometimes said to be a cause of ADD is hypoglycemia, which means low blood sugar. To a physician, hypoglycemia is not present unless the blood sugar drops below a certain level, and if the blood sugar is below that level, it may indicate some underlying disease or disorder. Hypoglycemia defined in this way is a very uncommon condition. When the blood sugar does drop below a certain level, most people will have odd feelings, including light-headedness, a feeling of weakness, irritability, a cold sweat, and palpitations. They often feel anxious. Only the irritability reminds one of the symptoms of ADD.

Despite the fact that hypoglycemia is uncommon, its diagnosis is frequently made. In many cases this is a mistake. The overdiagnosis of hypoglycemia may happen because some people experience mild changes, like those described above, when the blood sugar is low but still within the normal range. Some evidence suggests that experiencing these symptoms, even though the blood sugar is within normal range, occurs more frequently in people who are nervous or high strung. Since ADD children are frequently nervous and tense, that could explain why many people think that ADD children may have hypoglycemia. The idea that excess sugar causes behavioral problems is now receiving scientific attention. Experiments are being conducted along the same lines as in the food additive experiments. Children are being kept on a balanced diet and evaluated following the administration (without the knowledge of the children and their families) of either a large amount of sugar or an artificial sweetener. Thus far the results of these investigations have been negative. The children's behavior does not worsen to any appreciable degree when they receive sugar rather than sweetener, nor does their performance on appropiate psychological tests change.

If a parent thinks that his child experiences a worsening of behavior that seems related to what he eats, no harm will be done by altering the diet as long as the family pays attention to basic nutritional needs. Placing a child on a special diet may do real damage if that diet is deficient in essential nutrients. With regard to hypoglycemia in particular, it is wrong to assume without further investigation that the child has this medical condition.

Finally, some allergists have claimed that allergies to natural foods may cause ADD. Children with definite food allergies sometimes develop what is known as the tension-fatigue syndrome. In this condition, the child develops symptoms of excess fatigue (which may be accompanied by an increase in motor activity and restlessness), increased irritability, and a resulting increase in negative behavior. When the food allergy is appropriately treated—by eliminating the offending food from the diet—the child's behavior also improves. However, the behavior typical of the tension-fatigue syndrome bears only a superficial resemblance to attention deficit disorder. Though the child may be more restless and irritable, he doesn't have the other symptoms that go along with ADD. If the child already has ADD *and* in addition develops a food allergy with accompanying behavioral changes, this can be expected to make his ADD much worse. If the food allergy is treated, the ADD child's behavior should also improve, but his ADD problems will remain. Thus, although food allergy may worsen ADD in some cases, there is no evidence to suggest that allergies cause ADD.

Children with chronic hay fever also demonstrate behavioral changes when their hay fever is under poor control. They may become tired and irritable, with accompanying restlessness. Again, if the hay fever is successfully treated, their behavior often improves. Since hay fever is a common condition, many ADD children can be expected to have this allergy in addition to their ADD. If this is the case, treatment for the hay fever might be expected to help the child, but, again, it cannot be expected to eliminate completely his ADD problems.

I have emphasized the importance of physiological contributions to attention deficit disorder for two reasons. First, many people are unaware of them. Second, they are the most common causes of the problem. In a few instances, they play a minor role. The size of the physiological contribution can vary. In some children they are very large, and no matter how the children are raised problems will appear. In other children there are only slight physiological contributions. With these children, problems will be minor unless there are substantial family problems. In these instances one usually finds that the child has done reasonably well until serious family problems arose. Sometimes one cannot be sure of the origin of the child's difficulties since serious family tensions have been present at least since the time of the child's birth.

No matter how the ADD child's problems arise, they frequently lead to typical difficulties within the family. Some psychiatrists and psychologists see the family's stresses as being a cause of the ADD child's problems. Sometimes they are. Very often they are not but are instead understandable reactions to the burden of the child's unpredictable and difficult behavior.

Children, like adults, respond to distress in terms of their type of personality. ADD children react by being moody, naughty, restless. All families, of course, want to solve their internal problems; in families with ADD children, some resolution of such conflicts becomes even more important.

NATURE AND EFFECTS OF THE TEMPERAMENTAL PROBLEMS

In any given child it is impossible to say how much his personality and behavior are due to temperament (nature) and how much are the result of his life experience (nurture). By the time he is six or seven his temperament has affected his behavior, which in turn has affected others around him, and their reactions in turn have affected him. For example, an aggressive child (not necessarily an ADD child) will have bothered others, who in turn will have gotten angry, punished, and rejected him. The child feels rejected because he has been rejected (experience), but he has been rejected because he has been aggressive (temperament). Furthermore, a rejected child is more likely to feel frustrated and act aggressively. Temperament and experience snowball; they move in a vicious circle. The sorts of vicious circles that ADD children get into will be discussed presently.

The central inborn temperamental differences of ADD children include the following characteristic problems: (1) inattentiveness and distractibility, (2) impulsivity (the inability to inhibit oneself—to say "no" to oneself and follow through), (3) restlessness, (4) demandingness, (5) perceptual and learning difficulties, (6) social aggressiveness, and (7) hyperreactivity. These traits are biologically caused. They are *not* caused by the child's upbringing. However, these inborn traits affect experience and can also be affected by experience. The ways in which this can happen will be discussed below.

School Behavior

Although school problems were discussed in the previous chapter, they are so common and so important that it may be useful to explain again how they arise. To repeat, inattentiveness, distractibility, lack of stick-to-itiveness, and special learning difficulties (when present) interfere with academic progress despite the presence of a normal IQ. Even if the ADD child does not have special learning difficulties or perceptual problems, he will have a harder time learning than his intellectual peers. To learn, a child must tolerate frustration. Some subjects are hard to understand and cannot be mastered without stick-to-itiveness. To learn, a child must pay attention. Intelligence is not enough. If the child cannot pay attention to what is being taught, he is, for all practical purposes, not there. To learn, a child must have patience. Elementary school requires a good deal of (boring) repetition, practice, and drill. A child who cannot force himself to complete tedious, disagreeable school tasks will have trouble in mastering reading, spelling, and arithmetic. The ADD child is highly likely, therefore, to fall behind and become an underachiever. As the child falls further behind, he will experience more frustration and criticism from teachers, parents, and fellow students. His parents will nag him for not doing his homework. He may be placed in a catch-up class or a special learning disability class. He will regard himself as stupid and may be taunted as a "retard" by other children.

The problems of the ADD child change as he becomes older and progresses into advanced grades. Entry into junior high school amplifies his problems for several reasons. First, junior high school is less structured. The ADD child must monitor himself to be sure he goes where he is supposed to go at different times. Second, he has a number of different teachers. Since they know him less well than his elementary school teacher did, they are less likely to appreciate the possible strengths beneath his obvious weaknesses. Third, he begins to get homework that requires planning and application. No matter how smart he is, to be successful he must approach his homework systematically. In subjects requiring reading and outlining, he may be particularly handicapped. For all these reasons, if ADD persists, academic problems typically increase in junior high school. These realistic problems combined with the special psychological problems some ADD children develop in adolescence and with the psychological problems that often affect non-ADD adolescents can make the early teens a very difficult period for the ADD child.

Lack of success breeds low self-esteem and lack of enthusiasm. By the time the ADD youngster outgrows his distractibility and inattentiveness he may be so far behind and so soured on school that he only wants out.

Although he may now be "normal" physiologically and although the temperamental problems may have diminished or disappeared, he is so scarred by school that he has acquired a marked distaste for it and may even drop out.

Relationships with Other Children

Because of his bossiness, his teasing, his "play it my way or not at all" attitude, the ADD child is likely to be disliked by other children, and since he is not very sensitive to the feelings of others he may constantly do the wrong things. Even if he is not bossy, other problems associated with ADD may interfere with his peer relations. If the child is a boy and has coordination problems, the social problem will be worse. If he is chosen eighteenth when choosing up baseball teams, he will think little of himself. If, in addition, he has a temper tantrum when he strikes out, his popularity will not go up. In order to be liked he may resort to a number of maneuvers that will get him into trouble with both children and adults. He may boast, brag, lie, clown, or show off. As he gets older, he may try to prove his worth by doing the most dangerous, and most self-destructive, things: stealing, climbing to the highest place, and so forth. Note how the temperamental characteristics (demandingness, hyperreactivity) lead to experience (rejection) that can lead to misguided attempts to improve relationships; the resultant social complications may reinforce the low self-esteem and make social interaction even more difficult.

In his relationships with his brothers and sisters, the same temperamental problems lead to other social difficulties. All brothers and sisters are jealous of one another from time to time. The ADD child's behavior and the reactions that it produces in his parents predictably produce even more sibling envy and resentment than are common in any family. All the problems ordinarily associated with these sources of jealousies are aggravated and intensified. The ADD child's brothers and sisters are probably favored because they are "good children" and he is "bad." They get more praise, he gets more blame, and he is jealous of them. On the other hand, he receives more attention than they—

because he both demands it and requires it—and they may be jealous of him. Endless squabbling is often the result. Another, and unexpected, complication sometimes occurs if the ADD child is treated and improves. The "good" children start showing problems! There are two explanations for this: first, they may previously have had problems but no one had noticed because the ADD child's problems had been so much greater; second, the other children may have had no problems but have probably enjoyed their identification as the good children. When their ADD brother or sister improves, they lose their enviable position and then manifest behavior that is very similar to the reactions of a child when a brother or sister is born. They may become jealous, act immaturely, and demand more attention. Fortunately, this does not always happen. I mention it only because it is upsetting when it occurs unexpectedly and is less upsetting when one knows it can occur.

Relationships with Parents

The ADD child's relationship with his parents is burdened by the difficulties encountered throughout his development. Because of his temperamental problems, the ADD child tends to be unsatisfiable from infancy. The mother cannot stop his colic, cannot handle his sleep disturbances, cannot satisfy him or make him happy. As he grows older, his hyperreactivity, his impulsivity, and the other behavior problems I have discussed add tensions to family life. Nothing the parents seem to do helps very much or for very long. Probably the most common parental complaint is the difficulty in disciplining the ADD child. The child is inattentive and rapidly forgets. He is told to clean his room, but when he is half finished (or one-tenth finished), he starts doing something else. He is told not to jump down the stairs, stops for a while, and then impulsively does it again. He is not totally unresponsive to discipline. But he is much less responsive than non-ADD children. If parents are very firm and very consistent they will find the ADD child can be disciplined—at least to some extent. If they are not firm and not consistent, they may find that he is almost totally out of control. How he is handled will often (not always) make a large difference. This is obviously of great importance in management and will be discussed in the pertinent chapter.

The difficulty in controlling the ADD child's impulsivity has several disturbing effects. First, the child is a disappointment. Second, the child's chronic misbehavior is likely to make the parents angry. Third, the parents may see themselves as inept and inadequate. These feelings bring further emotional complications because the parents believe that they are not "supposed" to feel chronically angry toward their children. There are many emotions that people are not supposed to feel. One should not hate one's parents or one's child or envy one's sister. But such feelings do arise and, when they do, people tend to suppress them. They pretend they are not there, they ignore them, they refuse to acknowledge them. Usually people are successful in these attempts and most of the time they are unaware that these feelings exist. Every now and then, however, in everyone, such feelings break through. When they do, one usually feels bad and guilty. When the parents of the ADD child become aware of their angry feelings, they feel even more inadequate, and guilty and depressed as well. These feelings not only are highly distressing but also are likely to lead to techniques of child rearing that will aggravate the ADD child's problems. Since reward and punishment seem ineffective in discipline, the parents are already confused, frustrated, and baffled. The anger the child engenders may make the parents act with excessive harshness. They may remove bicycle or TV privileges for a week. They may spank the child a little too hard. The parents' awareness of their severity (to a small child!) tends to produce further guilt, which leads them to try to atone by being more lenient. Frequently this leads to a pattern of alternating excessive discipline and excessive permissiveness, a pattern that is the opposite of the consistent atmosphere in which the child functions best. The catch is that it is the child's behavior that is likely to make his parents behave inconsistently.

As a further complication, severe and harsh discipline (which is very different from firm discipline) can produce certain kinds of "problems," or maladjusted behavior, in *any* child, and these responses sometimes appear in the ADD child. Someone weak who feels he is being treated too harshly will feel resentful. But he has only limited ways of fighting back. He may comply resentfully, doing the job to the letter but not in the spirit of the law. He may merely pretend to comply. He may, at the risk of further punishment, dig in his heels and be negative, ornery, or stubborn. He may attempt to strike back by doing annoying, naughty, or hurtful things in another area. Nobody likes always being told what to do and what not to do. Even if the parent is a saint, the ADD child (who finds it difficult to inhibit himself) will feel as if he is receiving more than his share of dos and don'ts and will be more inclined to stiffen his back in protest.

This friction leads to problems in other areas. As the parent-child problems multiply, the ADD child will feel angry at his parents, but if one expresses anger at a loved one, one runs the risk of driving the loved one away. So in some cases the anger may not be expressed very directly. It can spill over and get taken out on a relatively innocent bystander, such as a playmate or teacher. The anger can also be completely bottled up. In adults this may be associated with psychosomatic disorders. For example, a person may keep his feelings inside himself but grow tense; in some instances he may actually get spasms and pains in his muscles (as expressed in the phrase "you give me a pain in the neck"). Lastly, the anger may be taken out on the child himself. This phenomenon is most surprising from the common-sense point of view but is frequently seen in very angry and inhibited adults. They will have accidents and hurt themselves; they will engage in behavior that results in humiliation or punishment. The same kind of behavior can sometimes be seen in the ADD child.

To further compound and complicate the difficulties, the child's behavior often causes disagreement and dispute between the parents. Both parents perceive the child as behaving poorly, and each tends to blame the other for disciplining or treating the child inadequately. In particular, the father is apt to notice that he is more effective in controlling the child. He is, of course, less frequently around the home, and when he appears he is likely to lower the boom, with the result that the child heaves to, at least briefly. The father's natural remark to his wife is: "I can control him—why can't you?" His wife, who spends much more time with the child, replies: "You can't treat him like that all day long," and the fight is on. Many parents have different views on how much strictness and severity are necessary in discipline. A parent whose own experience as a child has been with harsh discipline tends to favor this approach, and one whose experience has been gentler is likely to oppose it. Consequently, one sometimes sees the formation of family triangles. One parent will be cast in the role of the child's defender while the other becomes the prosecutor. The prosecutor parent, who is the odd man out, then has an additional problem. Not only does he (or she) have a difficult child, but also his (or her) spouse is siding with the child against him. The parent who has been pushed out then feels jealous of his own child. Again, jealousy is one of those feelings that parents are not "supposed" to have, but do. Brief reflection about one's own family or the families of friends should quickly bring to mind numerous illustrations of the complications, animosities, and guilt that can ensue.

Another and almost universal familial complication exists. In the recent past almost all child psychiatrists and psychologists have maintained that most of the behavioral problems seen in children were the results of the manner in which they were raised by their parents. Most parents who have done any reading on child rearing are aware of these notions but do not realize that they are becoming very much out of date. Such parents reach what they think is an obvious conclusion. They have a child with behavior difficulties. Children's behavior difficulties are the results of their parents' difficulties. Therefore, the parents—they themselves—must be either stupid or evil. Their child's difficulties are not only a serious problem in themselves but are also a reflection of the parents' failure as parents. Unfortunately, many mental health workers may reinforce the parents in this view. A substantial number of psychiatrists, psychologists, social workers, teachers, and school guidance counselors are unaware of the evidence for the physical basis of the problem of attention deficit disorder. They, too, believe that the child's problems are a reflection of his parents' problems. They will inform the parents, subtly or otherwise, that they are responsible for the child's difficulties. This will either intensify the parents' sense of guilt, anxiety, and depression, or lead them to deny that there is anything wrong with the child. The latter course would be difficult to follow, but rather than be labeled as bad parents of a bad child, some people will deny the evidence of their senses and proclaim that their child is perfectly normal but misunderstood by others. This is an understandable, common, and unfortunate technique that delays or prevents the problem from being solved. Many parents of ADD children have accused themselves for many years, and a final prosecution by experts may lead them to defend themselves by denying the existence of problems in the child, which in turn leads to the child's not receiving treatment. Contrary to usual belief, family disturbances are often the result and not the cause of a child's problems.

Certainly, these parent-child sequences are not seen in all families with ADD children and not even in most of them. They have been presented to illustrate how temperament in the child can produce changes in those around him, which in turn will produce psychological changes in the child. Notice that the temperament of the parent is very important in this equation. If the parent is hot-tempered or impulsive, because of either temperament or experience, he or she is more likely to become involved with and intensify the child's problems.

The Child's Feelings About Himself

Although the ADD child sometimes feels anger in response to his parents' reactions to his behavior, he more often has other reactive feelings that are more self-destructive. Because the child is rejected, criticized, and told he is exasperating, he will feel unlovable and unworthy and think little of himself. He is criticized by his teachers, who are likely to say, "You are bright enough to do better. . . . Why don't you try harder? . . . You could do better if you cared" (adding "like your brother or sister"—if they attended the same school). He is unpopular with his peers. They choose him less for games or not at all. He is not invited to parties or sleepovers. Because he is unpopular and highly reactive to teasing, he is frequently teased. His parents are usually exasperated. They continually express their annoyance, anger, or disappointment with him. Even if they do not openly compare him with his brothers and sisters, he can see that his parents like his siblings better. Parental self-control can diminish these feelings but it cannot prevent them. Even though he is somewhat thick-skinned and even though people may say nothing, the child cannot help noticing how they react to him.

Our self-esteem is formed on the basis of others' responses to us. We learn that we are attractive, nice, or bright, depending on whether others consider us good-looking, pleasant, and intelligent. The ADD child has a low opinion of himself. This is not neurotic; it is rational. He is failing at school, with his peers and with his parents. He fails in all the important areas of a child's life. He feels he is dumb, lazy, disobedient, and unlikable because that is the way his world regards him.

Obviously, anything that can help the child change his behavior will prevent him from suffering the consequences of that behavior. Although a child may eventually outgrow the physiological and the temperamental problems, the psychological difficulties he has had because of the temperamental problems may persist. He will have learned—and not forgotten—patterns of psychological maladjustment. On the other hand, if the physiological problems and symptoms can be kept in check until he outgrows them, he will avoid many bad experiences and grow up more easily. He will be better in school and have better relationships with his family and friends. He will not suffer severe consequences from his attention deficit disorder. Many ADD children can now be helped to achieve this major goal, as will be discussed in the chapter on treatment.

4

The Development of the Child with Attention Deficit Disorder

In the chapter on the characteristics of the ADD child, I discussed the changes in his problems as he grows. I also mentioned that the sequence of problems is not inevitable, and that many ADD children grow out of their problems as they become older. An obvious and reasonable question that the parents might ask is what the fate of their ADD child will be. This question is not easy to answer. The usual scientific way of replying to such a question is to look through the case records of people diagnosed as having the ailment several years ago, and then to evaluate the same patients at the present time. This procedure is difficult to follow with ADD since the syndrome has only recently begun to be widely recognized. If one does examine old records, one will not find children who have been diagnosed as ADD—or even as hyperactive. One will find children who one suspects would have been diagnosed as ADD if attention deficit disorder had been well known at that time. Since adequate old case records are not available, we will have to wait several years to see the developmental course of children who have currently been diagnosed as having ADD.

Nevertheless, we are not totally in the dark. We do have information from three sources. The first consists of psychiatrists who have been treating ADD (hyperactive) children for many years. The second consists of studies of severely disturbed children who were identified as hyperactive and labeled many years ago. The second source of information is likely to be misleading since it refers to a very small segment of ADD children, those whose problems were unusually severe.

We are beginning to obtain the best information from a third source—a few scientific studies, started several years ago, that were designed to explore systematically and to evaluate changes in the children that occurred over time.

Physicians who have treated hyperactive children over a period of years have repeatedly noted that in many of the children the problems tend to change, become less severe, and disappear with age. This sort of progress has caused some physicians to label the problem a developmental lag. (The implication is that the ADD child, who is immature, is like a child who is unusually short for his age. Both are likely to catch up, to become mature or taller, but later than most children.) In many ADD children some of the more troublesome symptoms gradually diminish and finally disappear around the time of puberty; in some children such improvements may occur earlier and in some later. In all ADD children some symptoms change and disappear. The ADD child may wet his bed longer than the nonhyperactive child, but he does not wet his bed forever. Similarly, restlessness and fidgetiness diminish with age. However—and this is extremely important—even though these symptoms may vanish, other ADD symptoms may persist. Difficulty in concentrating, lack of stick-to-itiveness, and impulsivity may remain. In talking to adults who had ADD problems in their youth one frequently hears that it was not until late adolescence or early adulthood that they finally settled down. Obvious hyperactivity disappeared whereas many of the other problems lingered for several years. Some adults continue to have ADD related problems. The practical consequence is that treatment, when effective, may need to be continued for several years after the most obvious and distressing symptoms have vanished.

In considering the practical implications of the development of the

ADD child, one must ask this question: "Is the persistence of symptoms due to the persistence of the temperamental (biochemical) problem, or is it due to maladjusted patterns of behavior that were learned because of the (no longer existing) temperamental problem?" The question cannot be answered in a general way, but a sensitive clinician can often give an approximate answer for an individual child. In some children, the problems do seem to persist because of the persisting temperamental difficulty. In other children the persistence of symptoms seems to be the result of behavior that was learned and now remains, so to speak, as a habit. (Similarly, a child who had broken his right arm and learned to write with his left hand might well retain indefinitely the ability to write with his left hand even after the fracture healed.) Some persisting symptoms were originally considered psychological but now seem of possible physiological origin. For example, when ADD drug treatment is given for the first time to adults in their thirties and forties with ADD-like symptoms, they sometimes demonstrate organizational abilities they never knew they had (accompanied by an increase in self-esteem).

The temperamental difficulty often responds well to medical treatment. This will be discussed in the next chapter. Learned behavior is not so easy to change, particularly if it is learned in early life. For example, children exposed to a foreign language before they are five or six learn it more easily and remember more of it than does an intelligent adult. Habits and attitudes, like skills, are learned more quickly and better when young, and habits learned when young are harder to unlearn. Further, some personality traits and attitudes developed in adolescence can be very durable, so it is desirable that the child have every physical and psychological advantage as he approaches that period. For example, in one study thin women who had been fat in childhood or in adolescence were asked how they regarded themselves. Interestingly, only those women who had been fat in adolescence had suffered psychological effects and continued to regard themselves as unattractive despite the fact that they were thin. Attitudes learned during the teen-age years had stuck with them. The relevance for ADD children is, I hope, obvious. The sooner that maladaptive learning can be prevented, the better, for the child will have less difficulty in adolescence and later life than he would have otherwise. If such habits or attitudes are learned, the outlook is not grim. Learned habits can be unlearned, skills can be acquired, and new experiences can change personality throughout one's life. The chapter on treatment will consider some psychological approaches that are pertinent here. But from what we know about children's growth and development, *early prevention would seem to be more effective than later treatment.*

When ADD symptoms persist to a significant degree into adolescence, special issues arise because the ADD problems interact with the normal psychological changes that occur when a child is undergoing adolescence.

From school age on, children's peers play an increasingly large role in their social development. As children enter adolescence the impact of their friends becomes even greater. Distraught parents are frequently aware that their adolescent child adopts values of his peer group that are in opposition to previously accepted home values. The adolescent is strongly motivated to form close relationships with his peers. Intimacy with equals replaces intimacy with parents. Adolescents confide in each other but often mumble or are mute with their parents.

Forming relationships with peers is sometimes a problem for the pre-adolescent ADD child. For the ADD adolescent who continues to lack social perceptiveness and skill, problems with peers continue. If his ADD handicaps affect the kinds of talents that make adolescents popular—for example, if he is poorly coordinated in athletic performance—he is additionally limited in making close friends. The lack of peer acceptance in adolescence is even more painful than it is in childhood.

Many ADD children seem to get less pleasure from the activities that other children enjoy. They may require excitement and dangerous situations to experience the pleasure that other children derive from less stimulating activities. The search for excitement increases the possibility that the ADD adolescent may associate with delinquent peers. A tendency toward depression (both in reaction to difficulties resulting from ADD and perhaps as a part of the ADD itself) may also play a role in excitement seeking. The combination of continuing low self-esteem (amplified by peer rejection), impaired social skills, and impulsivity may lead the child to associate with any group of fellows who accept him, including those engaged in delinquent activities.

One of the major areas of psychological growth in adolescents is development of autonomy—feelings of self-sufficiency and freedom from one's parents. This is a healthy pattern, even if it causes temporary conflict between parents and adolescent. The severity of the conflict may depend on how the adolescent expresses increasing autonomy. Preferences for current adolescent fashions in music, hair styles, and clothing may produce mild parental irritation, but idealistic or activist political positions at variance with parental ones, or becoming a member of a social outgroup, can result in serious disruption of family bonds.

Another important adolescent developmental task is establishing precourtship relationships with the opposite sex, which requires social ease and social skills. Because of his social obtuseness, the ADD adolescent may not be shy, but because of his social ineptitude, he stands a good chance of being unsuccessful.

Still another area—most conspicuous in those who showed insufficient conscience as children—is continuing problems with self-control. Self-control involves a number of psychological attributes that ADD adolescents tend to be deficient in: control of impulsivity; empathy; ability to perceive one's effect on others. These deficits contribute to social immaturity and increase the possibility that the ADD adolescent will become involved in delinquent acts.

Recently, a number of us who are doing continuing research in this field have discovered that in some unfortunate persons many ADD problems persist until the thirties or forties. We first became aware of this in talking to the parents of ADD children. Frequently, the parents mentioned that they had been hyperactive in childhood and that the problems had become less severe with age but still bothered them to an annoying degree. These adults differed from ADD children not only in that many of the problems were less severe than they had been, but also in that the parents had developed adult ways of coping with their problems. Of particular interest—and practical importance—was our discovery that many of the adults who continued to suffer from ADD problems could benefit from treatment with medications as much as ADD children.

Similarly, "learning disabilities" may persist well into the thirties and forties. Although *apparently* (there is no really substantial information) spurts naturally occur at around age eight and in the early teens, during which learning disabilities improve, there is an overall tendency for learning disabled children to fall further and further behind with age. Perhaps one-third of learning disabled children continue to have serious problems well into adult life. In the other two-thirds some improvement occurs, but learning disabled children often continue to be slow readers and poor spellers, and, if they have had difficulty with arithmetic, they continue to have problems in performing arithmetical calculations.

The above statements may be disheartening. However, early and well-administered psychological treatment, in combination with appropriate medication if indicated, may prevent—or greatly reduce—the psychological symptoms that develop on the basis of the physiological abnormalities. Such treatment, of course, does not cure the underlying physiological abnormalities, and perhaps the reason that some treatment programs in the past proved ineffective may simply be that they did not administer medication long enough. Without treatment, the number of children who continue to have problems is larger than was previously believed. Since we now have evidence that some ADD children continue to have the same physiological difficulties in adult life (inattentiveness, hot temper, not being able to complete tasks, and so on) and continue to respond to medication, it seems obvious that some ADD children may benefit from—and may need to take—medicine for many years after childhood.

The developmental picture that I have been discussing has emerged largely from reports by physicians with extensive clinical experience with a great range of hyperactive children, and from new scientific studies. The other major source of information—old studies of severely disturbed hyperactive children—is not very illuminating with regard to most ADD children since it deals with those few whose difficulties are profound. These studies have shown that seriously disturbed hyperactive children are more likely to have serious psychiatric disorders in later life. It is obvious that this small group of children should receive continuing treatment from an early age.

At this point, and almost as an aside, another remark should be made about brain damage and ADD. As emphasized, documented brain damage is not the cause of most cases of ADD. When brain damage is related to ADD, it generally appears to be damage sustained around the time of birth or during pregnancy. At present we do not know if the subgroup of ADD children who do have such damage are subject to a developmental course that is different from that experienced by other ADD children. Most people regard brain injury as permanent and irreversible, but this is because our usual experience is with brain injury in adults. There are differences in the effects of such injury at different periods of life, however. It might be reassuring to mention some of the things that are known about the effects of brain injury in very early life. The most important fact is that brain development often compensates for very early injury. Although the young, like the old, cannot grow new brain cells, they sometimes can adjust to brain injury quite well, apparently because the functions of the damaged areas are taken over by other portions of the brain. This can be illustrated by some experiments on monkeys. If a certain part of the brain of an *adult* monkey is removed he will behave as if he had a stroke: one side of his body will be paralyzed (or weak) and uncoordinated. If the same portion of an *infant* monkey is removed he will have difficulties at first but over time he will recover complete function: he will not be weak or uncoordinated on one side of his body. Obviously, there are no similar experiments on children but the implication is clear. One can hope for more recovery from an injury in the young than from the same injury in the old.

To summarize, first, at least half of ADD children (and possibly more), particularly those whose symptoms are not severe, outgrow their symptoms at or around the time of puberty. Second, about 25 to 30 percent of ADD children lose some of their symptoms at puberty but may continue to have other symptoms for several years thereafter. Sometimes these ADD-like symptoms are actually the customary adjustment problems that males experience in adolescence. In the remaining 10 to 25 percent of ADD children, the picture of later development is mixed and unclear. All these children *may* suffer some psychological effects from their temperamental problems, and treatment should be considered for them at least until they outgrow the temperamental symptoms.

Finally, in some ADD children, the problems of inattentiveness, impulsivity, and even hyperactivity persist into adulthood. Recognition of these possibilities is important for diagnosis and correct treatment. I will discuss what is now known about ADD in adults in a later chapter.

5

Treatment of the Child with Attention Deficit Disorder

The treatment of the ADD child is often relatively simple. Since medication is of the greatest importance, treatment almost always requires the services of a physician. Nonmedical specialists, such as psychologists, educators, and social workers may provide useful and sometimes absolutely necessary assistance, but in most instances they cannot assume primary responsibility for treatment. Since they are not trained to use and cannot prescribe medications, they are unable to supply the treatment that is both the best and sometimes the only treatment required. This must be emphasized because too often the ADD child or his family is referred to a psychologist, social worker, or school guidance counselor. Such referrals are made because of psychological maladjustment in the child, problems in the family, or failure in school. These problems, as I have said, may be a result of ADD in the child, and they may also worsen ADD in the child. Some, particularly family problems, may be largely irrelevant.

What frequently happens is that the ADD child is misdiagnosed and referred for help, and it is then noticed that his parents have marital problems. Someone then assumes that the child's problems are the result of family problems, and the parents receive treatment. This happens frequently because the traditional view in child psychiatry has been that most children's problems are the product of their parents' or their families' problems. The difficulty is that a large number of married couples have serious problems. An increasingly large proportion of all marriages end in divorce. Of those that do not, perhaps half have serious difficulties. Thus, the chances are great that the parents of any child are having difficulties. If one looked at the parents of children with rheumatic fever, epilepsy, or mental retardation, one would find that the majority of them had marital problems. (And, in fact, some of these problems might be caused by the child's illness.) No one would expect that helping the parents would cure a child's rheumatic fever, epilepsy, or mental retardation. Helping the parents might, and probably would, make the child happier. Similarly, it is quite possible that the parents of an ADD child are having marital difficulties; if one helps only the parents, the child will probably be more comfortable in some ways, but his basic problems will remain untouched and unchanged. A major difficulty for the ADD child is that his problems are often not recognized as medical. His medical problems manifest themselves in his behavior, and until recently all such problems were thought to be psychologically caused. The reasoning has been that if he has psychological problems, his parents, and perhaps he himself, require only psychological treatment. Simple—and very incorrect. Normal children may have disturbed parents. Disturbed children may have normal parents. Disturbed children may have disturbed parents and the two sets of disturbances may be largely separate.

The same observations that apply to psychological help for family problems apply in part to the individual psychological treatment of the ADD child, or child psychotherapy. Almost all ADD children have psychological problems. *Sometimes* these can be helped by psychotherapy. But as long as the temperamental problems remain, the psychological problems will continue to spring up. In other words, the young ADD child—and the adolescent child in whom temperamental problems remain—will require treatment for those temperamental problems. Psychotherapy may benefit the child—and later I will discuss how—but unless he is medically treated it is very likely that he will develop new problems.

Finally, the same principles hold for educational treatment. The school counselor will see the child with educational problems or behavioral problems or both. He may assume that the behavioral problems are causing the academic ones, or that the academic problems are causing the behavioral problems. He is probably *partly* right in either case. The catch is that both kinds of problems can be separately caused by ADD. Dealing with either without treating the underlying disorder may be helpful but it is not the best treatment.

To repeat, the help provided by trained professionals other than physicians can be important and sometimes necessary to the ADD child and his family, but most ADD children require medical treatment; at present only physicians are in a position to provide such treatment. Once the child has embarked on the basic course of medical treatment, it will be easier to decide whether the parents should also seek help for him from a psychologist, social worker, or teacher.

All three major forms of treatment will be discussed in this chapter: medical, psychological, and educational. I will also add a few words about help for the youngster whose ADD is discovered in adolescence.

MEDICAL TREATMENT

A very large fraction of ADD children can be helped, often to a marked degree, by treatment with medication. In some children this may be the *only* treatment that is required. In others psychological and educational treatment may also be necessary. It is often difficult beforehand to determine how much of a child's trouble is caused by family difficulties and how much by his own temperament. Often, after a child has been treated with medications some of the problems may disappear while others will remain. The physician may then suggest psychological treatment for the family and/or the child and/or educational treatment for the child.

The use of medication to treat children is sometimes upsetting to parents. Parents are troubled for various reasons and it may be useful to discuss them.

First, many parents have difficulty coming to terms with the fact that their child's behavior problems have a physical rather than a psychological basis; often this is because they find physical problems frightening. They feel that in the area of behavior what is psychological can easily be remedied whereas what is physical cannot. They feel that a temper tantrum is soon over, but the damaged brain may never recover. For this reason they would rather believe that the problem is psychological. If the child's misbehavior is psychological, surely the powerful psychiatrists can change it, but how can his brain be cured? On both counts the parents' information is incomplete. Fortunately, just as with many other serious physical problems, behavior malfunctions with physical origins can sometimes be easiy remedied. On the other hand, psychological treatment is by no means as effective as it is sometimes believed to be. Certain common forms of brain tumor that cause profound psychological disturbances can be easily removed, whereas, in contrast, some neuroses of psychological origin cannot be cured despite years of expensive and time-consuming psychological treatment. Pneumonia can often be cured with a single shot of penicillin. Pernicious anemia, formerly a fatal disease, can be completely cured by vitamin administration. But a child who has been neglected and psychologically abused during early childhood may never function normally even if he later receives warm, considerate parental care and psychotherapy.

A second reason parents sometimes object to treatment with medication is that treatment with medication seems artificial. To many parents it does not appear to be a good way to discover the root of the problem. That may be so if the root of the problem is psychological, but in this case it is generally physical. Because some regulatory functions of the brain are operating less efficiently than usual, chemical means must be used to improve their functioning. Medication can be looked on as a form of replacement therapy; that is, it apparently supplies chemicals that are lacking or causes the body to create more of the missing chemicals. At present, we can give no chemical that will permanently cure the deficiency. Unlike pneumonia, attention deficit disorder has no one-shot cure. Medication is necessary until the brain, through its own growth and development, begins producing adequate amounts of the required chemicals. This is very similar to the treatment required for pernicious anemia, except that the pernicious anemia requires administration of vitamin B_{12} throughout the patient's life; unlike the patient with pernicious anemia, the ADD child sometimes outgrows his difficulties.

A third reason parents sometimes object to medication is that they fear the child will become dependent on it. By dependency, parents generally mean two things. First, they fear that the medication is related to the substances currently feared as drugs. They sometimes fear that, like the drug addict, the child will feel so good after taking the medication that he will become addicted to it. This is never true of the medications employed by physicians in the treatment of ADD. Children may be happy about the improvement in their lives that medicine helps to produce but they never like the medicine. They do not get high from it. They don't get kicks from it. Medically, any non-naturally occurring substance that is administered to a person with the hope of therapeutic results is a drug. Aspirin is a drug. So is penicillin. Certain forms of hormones are drugs. The problem is not whether a substance is a medication or a drug but whether it is beneficial or harmful. As will be seen, most of the medications used in the treatment of ADD are beneficial and carry very little risk.

A second form of dependency that parents sometimes fear is the need for constant medication to handle problems. In this respect the parents are correct, but the dependency is preferable to the ailment. Many ADD children do need medicine to control their problems. The ADD child is in a position similar to but less threatening than that of the child with diabetes, epilepsy, or rheumatic fever. Children with those disorders must take insulin, anti-epileptic drugs, or penicillin for the rest of their lives. The ADD child may be luckier. Since well over half of ADD children outgrow their symptoms, the ADD child may have to take medication for only a part of his life.

In discussing the major medications employed by most physicians in the treatment of ADD children, their effects, and their administration, my aim will be to help the parent understand the physician's treatment goals. I will not be presenting an exhaustive list of medications, and of course the discussion is not intended to enable parents to treat their child by themselves. Parents who are aware of how a drug should act, what side effects it can produce, and what (if any) possible hazards accompany its use are in a much better position to assist their physicians in the treatment of their child. With this in mind, let us now turn to some general aspects of the administration of medication to ADD children.

The first very important point to be made is that several medications are potentially helpful for children with ADD. It is impossible to predict how a child will respond to a particular medication. Some children respond very well to one medication and not to another. It may be necessary to try several before the best one is found.

Sometimes the medication does not take effect immediately but seems to require a cumulative buildup in the body, so that it is necessary for a child to be on the medicine for some time before one can decide how effective it can be. This period may be as long as several weeks. In a few instances the medicine will at first seem to make the child's symptoms worse; parents should be aware of this so that they will not stop the medication immediately. In these few instances, after a week or two of deterioration, a child's symptoms and problems may then begin to get better.

Another important principle is that in beginning any course of medication the physician will start at the smallest dose that is ever effective, since he does not wish to give more medication than is necessary. Because of this, it is often necessary to increase the amount of medicine considerably. This should be no cause for alarm. Children differ greatly, and some children need much larger amounts of medication than others. The amount of medication is not necessarily related to the seriousness of the problem. For example, some extremely hyperactive children require only very small amounts of medicine whereas some children who are much less hyperactive need larger amounts.

Many medications produce side effects. A side effect is an undesired by-product of the administration of medicine. For example, aspirin sometimes produces irritation of the lining of the stomach and mild abdominal pain. Antihistamines, given for hay fever, sometimes cause sleepiness. The medications used in treating ADD children will sometimes produce side effects. When I discuss the individual medications, I will mention these side effects.

Lastly, all medicines (including aspirin and penicillin) may produce allergic reactions. An allergic reaction occurs only in a small proportion of people who receive medication. Some medications are much more likely to produce allergies than others. The drugs most commonly used in treating ADD children, the stimulant drugs, very rarely produce allergies. Some medications that are used when the stimulant drugs do not seem to be the best treatment for an individual child are somewhat more likely to produce allergies. The parents should know the symptoms of allergies and should contact the doctor if they do occur. Although this rarely happens, if allergies are allowed to go on, they sometimes become worse. Some major symptoms are quite obvious: skin rash, hives, etc. One other major symptom that many people are not aware of is a decrease in white blood cell count, which results in an increased susceptibility to infections. When such an allergy occurs it is most common for a person to develop a sore throat and a high fever. Of course, most children who are not receiving medications of any sort occasionally get sore throats and high fevers, but a child who is receiving medication and develops such symptoms should immediately be seen by a physician.

Stimulant Drugs

The medications most frequently used in the treatment of ADD children are the stimulant drugs. The most common of these are d-amphetamine (several trade names, of which perhaps the most common is Dexedrine) and methylphenidate (trade name: Ritalin). Amphetamine was first used for the treatment of ADD children in 1937. Methylphenidate has been used since the early 1960s. A less common drug, pemoline (trade name: Cylert), was available in Europe for a number of years before its relatively recent introduction into the United States. These are generally the most effective and safest medicines available in the treatment of ADD children. Approximately two-thirds of ADD children respond well to one of these drugs. Although the drugs are about equal in effectiveness, a particular child may respond better to one than to another. If one drug provides only moderate improvement or produces annoying side effects, a physician may then try another.

Despite their effectiveness and safety, amphetamines and methyl-phenidate have recently acquired a bad repuation because they may cause adults to become high and psychologically dependent on them. (Amphetamine is well known as speed.) Pemoline does not appear to have this property, and, although it has been available in Europe for some time, little or no abuse has occured. However, like the amphet-amines and methylphenidate, it is stimulating to normal adults. Stim-ulant drugs have a much different effect in ADD children than they do in normal adults. Rather then becoming high or excited, ADD children are in general calmed down by these drugs and sometimes (rarely) they may even become somewhat sad. Children do not become addicted to these medications; there is absolutely no danger that this will occur. If the ADD child's problems persist into adolescence, many physicians will discontinue the use of the stimulant drugs and substitute medications that are not habit-forming in adults. However, many physicians who have treated numerous ADD children may continue to use the stimulant drugs well into adolescence—with caution—because of their medical impression that these children do not begin to respond to the drugs as do normal adults until they have outgrown their ADD problems.

The ADD adults I have treated so far—and their number is still small—have generally shown the same response to medication that ADD children do. They become, as I discuss further below, calm rather than excited, and they do not get high. Furthermore, the ADD adults I have treated continue to benefit from the same relatively small doses. This contrasts with adults who abuse stimulant drugs for their pleasant effects, who must escalate the dosage, sometimes to a hundred times as much, to continue to receive the drug effect.

Effects

When the stimulant drugs are effective, ADD children generally become calmer and less active, develop a longer span of attention, become less stubborn, and are easier to manage (they "mind" better). In addition, they frequently become more sensitive to the needs of others and much more responsive to discipline. Frequently, fuses are lengthened and temper tantrums become fewer or disappear. Mood may stabilize, impulsivity decrease, handwriting improve, and the child may become less disorganized. When stimulants work the child matures and may function better—at least temporarily—than he has ever functioned in his life. The response of the ADD child to stimulant medication is unlike any other medication response in psychiatry. At best, most other treatments restore a patient to his previous level of functioning. The temporary psychological growth that occurs when stimulants are effective is very different from simple slowing down or quieting. And it is a very different effect from that which the parent—if he does not have ADD—may have experienced with tranquilizers or stimulants. Tranquilizers and stimulants used by adults respectively slow down and relax, and rev up. They do not stabilize mood, cool tempers, make one more law-abiding, dampen impulsivity, and help one to plan ahead.

The widespread effect of stimulant medication on various psychological functions has led child psychiatrists to believe that the brain chemistry of people with ADD is in some ways different from that of others. The medication seems to compensate at a basic level for this chemical difference, affecting behavior in many diverse areas. It should be emphasized that these effects are very different from those of the so-called tranquilizing drugs. Tranquilizing drugs may slow a child down but they do not increase his attention span, personal sensitivity, or reasonableness.

When the stimulant drugs are effective, they produce one of the most dramatically effective responses that can be seen in psychiatry. If the child is responsive to amphetamines and methylphenidate, the medications are usually effective immediately. In a few instances, the effects described may take as long as a week or two to appear. The effects of pemoline are seen much more slowly; it may take two or three weeks for pemoline's full benefit to be realized. As mentioned, occasionally a child taking stimulant drugs will appear to be worse at first—he may become more irritable and more active. In quite a few (not all) of these cases, if he continues to receive medication, this effect goes away and he becomes calmer.

Dosage

Parents' evaluation of their child's adjustment will play an important role in the doctor's decision to increase or decrease the dose of the medication. The parents should know something about the dosages ordinarily employed. Medications are usually measured in milligrams. A milligram (one-thousandth of a gram) is a unit of weight, about 1/30,000th of an ounce. The amount of dextroamphetamine (*d*-amphetamine) an ADD child may require usually ranges from about 5 to 60 milligrams a day. The amount of methylphenidate an ADD child may require ranges from 10 to 120 milligrams a day. Pemoline, which comes in odd dosages, is usually prescribed in amounts between 18.75 and 112.5 milligrams per day. There are occasional exceptions, in either direction: a very few children will require less than these dosages, and a few will require more.

Dextroamphetamine is available in two forms: tablets and long-acting capsules. The tablets generally last from 3 to 6 hours, whereas the long-acting form of the medicine lasts anywhere from 8 to 16 hours. Unfortunately, in some brands the release of medication is not gradual and even. The capsules or tablets may release too much medication initially, followed by too little over time. The patient gets too large a dose at first, followed by too low a dose thereafter. Methylphenidate is available as tablets whose effects are somewhat shorter, perhaps lasting 3 to 4 hours. For this reason it is often given two or three times a day (morning, noon, and perhaps early afternoon). Recently, a long-acting form of methylphenidate, Ritalin-SR, has been introduced. The manufacturers had hoped that it would remain active for as long as 8 hours and that it would have to be given only once or twice a day. This seems to work with some children but not with others, so that the drug must be given more than twice a day. Another disadvantage is that it is available only in 20-milligram form, which makes fine tuning of dosage impossible when it is used alone. The duration of action of pemoline varies. In some children it must be given twice a day while in others it appears to last approximately 12 to 18 hours; in a few its effects *perhaps* may carry over to the next day and even longer. The advantage of the long-acting forms of medication is that the child receives medication only once a day, in the morning; in contrast, the tablets usually have to be given two or three times a day. For the reasons mentioned above, however, the use of the long-acting forms of medication is not always possible.

If the child is taking a medication whose effects last only 3 or 4 hours, and does not come home from school for lunch, the medication must be administered around noon at school. In some schools the nurse can do this, although many children do not want to visit the nurse because they are afraid the other children will identify them as being different. This is particularly so when teachers tell the child in front of the class that he should take his behavior medicine. It is easy to see that under these circumstances, a child may become negativistic about taking medication at all. Many children assume responsibility themselves for taking their medicine at school. The task is easiest if the child brings his lunch to school rather than buying it in the cafeteria. The medication can be wrapped separately—for example, in a small piece of aluminum foil—and packed with a sandwich. The drug can also be carried in a pocket, but if the child is a chronic forgetter, it may be impossible to use short-acting drugs such as methylphenidate. In such instances, one may have to switch to long-acting drugs such as dextroamphetamine or pemoline (if there are no contraindications to their use, as described below).

It is important for parents to realize that the effects of stimulant drugs (with the possible exception of pemoline) last for only a brief period of time. For the amphetamines and methylphenidate there is no carryover and for pemoline there is generally no carryover from one day to the next. When the medication is effective, the parents will find that if it is discontinued for a day, the child's temperamental problems promptly reappear. Thus, the child's ADD problems may be present in the morning until he receives his medication. If part of his problem is dawdling about getting dressed, eating breakfast, and going to school, it may be useful or necessary to give him the medication as soon as he awakens. Similarly, the effect of the medicine will wear off as the day goes on. If the medicine wears off at three or four o'clock and a parent's main contacts with the child are only after he comes home from school, the parent may get the impression that the medicine is not helping. To check up on this, the parent should carefully observe the child's behavior on the weekend, at times when the medicine is most active— that is, mornings and early afternoons. This will also allow the parent to observe carefully how long each dose lasts and help the doctor to determine the best spacing of doses. Since the medicines are generally given in doses that permit the effects to wear off in the late afternoon or early evening, parents may anticipate more difficulty with the child at that time. If they are planning to take the child out in the evening or, say, to attend a large family gathering, it is often helpful to give a small additional dose later in the afternoon. As a rule this is not done routinely because these drugs tend to keep children awake.

After beginning with the smallest dose of medication that has been found useful with ADD children, the physician will then usually follow the principle of increasing the medication until either the child's behavioral problems improve to what seems to be the greatest possible extent, or the side effects of increased dosages cause a problem in themselves.

In order to determine how much benefit the child is receiving, the physician will want to know what is happening at home and at school. The schoolteacher is in an excellent position to determine the effects of medicine because of seeing the child in a circumstance in which he is apt to have the most difficulty. Furthermore, the teacher can compare his behavior with that of many other children of his age and intellectual ability. It is an excellent idea for the parent to stay in regular contact with the teacher whenever the medication is being adjusted or changed. The parent should tell the teacher that the child is receiving treatment and should ask for a report on any changes the teacher may notice in the child's classroom behavior. Practically, it is useful not to make a big issue about this kind of information. Most people who expect to find changes tend to see them even if they are not present, so the parent should merely request information and not suggest that the teacher should expect to see the child improve. Another reason for not suggesting that the child may improve is that many teachers, trying to spare parents' feelings, will fail to report any difficulty the child may be having in school. If the child improves somewhat, and is now only a minor problem rather than a major problem, the teacher may inform the parent that things are going "pretty well." What the parent wants to know is if there are any problems, what kind they are, and how bad they are.

When the medicine is given depends on the sorts of problems the ADD child has. If they occur primarily in school, many physicians will prescribe the medicine only during the school week and not on weekends, holidays, and vacations. If there are problems both at school and at home, the physician will recommend that the medication be given every day. After the medicine has been taken for some time most physicians like to employ vacations from therapy or medication-free periods. This is done for two reasons. The first is to give the child a rest from medicine. Although there is no evidence that these medications are harmful, most physicians would prefer to give as little as possible of any medicine. A second reason for rest periods is to see if the child has outgrown his need for the medication. Often, as the child grows older, he will need the medication only during his stressful periods. That means that the medication can be stopped during school vacations. As the child becomes still older, the physician may want the child to begin school in the fall without medication and see how he does through the first few weeks. During this time the parents should, of course, stay in close touch with the school to see if problems are developing. If no problems emerge, that will provide considerable evidence that the ADD child is outgrowing his problems. As discussed before, the parents should always bear in mind that hyperactivity and restlessness them-selves may disappear, whereas other problems, such as poor concen-tration and underachievement, may persist. The parents should therefore request detailed information from the teacher. Information that the child is not restless is not sufficient. How he is adjusting with his classmates, how he is concentrating on his tasks, and how much work he is able to do and how well must all be examined closely.

The purpose of giving medication is more than simply to control the child's behavior and allow him to adjust to an environment he does not like and in which he does poorly: school. Effective medication often affords the child self-control. In a sense he will have more, not less freedom, and will suffer less from symptoms such as moodiness and anger. By being less bossy, more obedient (but he does not become a robot!), cooler tempered, and a better student, he will be better liked by teachers, parents, siblings, and peers. He will feel better about himself and about his life. More than his school performance improves. His life improves.

A final point. Unlike adults, children generally do *not* become tolerant to the effects of these medications, although it is common to see a small amount of tolerance develop during the first few weeks of treatment. In those instances one finds that a dosage of medication that for a month or so provided relief of symptoms gradually fails to control those symptoms. The physician will then usually increase the medication and find no further development of tolerance. Usually, if a child stays on the medication for several years, he will require an increased dose of medication as he becomes older and larger. In a few instances children do become tolerant to one of the stimulant drugs. In such circumstances most physicians then switch to another drug. Occasionally, it is necessary to alternate drugs in this manner. If the development of a drug tolerance continues to present a problem, the physician will often then switch to still another of the major categories of medications that are used.

Side effects

When given to children, the stimulant drugs are unusually safe medications. Because the stimulants have opposite effects in children and adults (as noted, adults are made high and excited; children are not and often are made calm), the effect of these medications is sometimes called paradoxical. This is true only in some respects and not in others. In both children and adults the stimulant drugs decrease appetite and tend to interfere with sleep. Usually the child's appetite returns after a while. Occasionally, the effect on appetite continues and is accompanied by some degree of weight loss. Although this weight loss may produce some concern in the parents, it never occurs to a medically serious degree. (Children's appetite generally returns in the evening after the medication wears off. Accordingly, they should be allowed to eat after supper and as much as they like. Appetite will also be normal, of course, at breakfast, before the medication has had time to act.) The drug's tendency to keep some children awake can usually be controlled by careful administration. Medication keeps children awake only while it is still in the bloodstream (that is, 3 to 6 hours after the last dose of pills and up to 18 to 24 hours for the long-acting capsules). This is the reason for *not* giving these medications late in the day. If sleeplessness continues to be a problem, it can generally be handled by *not* using the long-acting form of the medicine but by using pills instead and by being careful not to give the last pill too late in the day. When the medication is adjusted this way, sleeplessness will not be a problem. However, behavior problems may appear later in the day as the medication wears off. If this constitutes a substantial problem, the physician may suggest the use of a sedative major tranquilizer (thioridazine—Mellaril—is the one generally employed) at bedtime. These drugs chemically block the arousing effects of stimulants and thus allow the child to fall asleep.

Allergies to the amphetamines and methylphenidate are very rare. Approximately 1 to 2 percent of children receiving pemoline will develop an allergy to the medicine. The allergy is not evident from symptoms such as skin rash but can be detected initially only by means of blood tests. Because some children do become allergic to pemoline and because it can only be detected in its early stages by blood tests, children receiving pemoline must have such blood tests every few months. In the event that allergy develops, pemoline must be discontinued. So far as is known, there are usually no long-term ill effects after discontinuation.

Stimulant medications and growth

Several years ago a report was published stating that stimulant medications decreased the rate of growth of both height and weight in ADD children. Since that report appeared, a number of other studies on the same subject have been published. It does appear that growth rate is slowed for a period of one or two years. After that, growth rate appears to approach normal. The whole issue is complicated because ADD children may have growth patterns that are different from those of other children and the usual tables of growth may not apply to ADD children. Doctors who have treated ADD children with stimulants from childhood through adolescence have not observed any long-term effects of stimulant medication on height. When slowing of growth velocity occurs, this trend can be changed by the use of lower doses of medication and summer vacations from medicine. Research is being conducted to determine the exact effects of stimulant medication on growth.

There is no doubt that many ADD children do lose weight on stimulant medication. Although this is sometimes upsetting to parents, there is no information suggesting that it is harmful, and apparently weight returns to normal when the medication is stopped. I should reemphasize that the effects that have been reported are small and that most physicians treating ADD children regard the psychological benefits as outweighing *possible* effects on the rate of growth. At a practical level, what the physician must do is follow the child's height, weight, and changes in adjustment, and base the use of stimulant medication not only on its effect on growth but on its effects on the child's psychological well-being.

Major Tranquilizers

Another group of medications sometimes used in the treatment of attention deficit disorder consists of the so-called major tranquilizers. Currently, they are rarely employed. Their major use is in counteracting the effects of stimulants and preventing insomnia, and in helping to control aggressive ADD children or ADD children who also have other psychiatric problems. These medications, first discovered about thirty years ago, have been used in the treatment of serious psychiatric disorders in adults. They are sometimes employed when the stimulant drugs are ineffective, and are sometimes extremely effective. They are absolutely nonhabit-forming or addicting, and with certain precautions are very safe. There are literally dozens of them, and many are very similar chemically. They are also very similar in their effects, with some slight differences that make now one, now another, desirable for an individual child. Those most generally employed, and this list is far from complete, are: chlorpromazine (Thorazine), thioridazine (Mellaril), trifluoperazine (Stelazine), haloperidol (Haldol). Sometimes physicians will recommend still other compounds if for some reason those most commonly used seem undesirable in a particular instance.

Effects

When these medications are effective, children gradually become less anxious, quieter, and easier to live with and manage. The medications have two effects. At first they tend to produce sleepiness, but after several days or weeks, the sleepy (or groggy) feelings usually disappear. The sleep-producing quality of the medicine is not what is being sought, but in order to obtain the useful tranquilizer effects one must put up with the sleepiness for a while. In general, they do not increase attention span, decrease stubbornness, stabilize mood, or help the child to organize himself. They may decrease impulsivity and temper outbursts.

Dosage

The doses of different tranquilizing medications vary considerably. For example, chlorpromazine is usually given in amounts ranging from about 30 to 600 milligrams a day. Haloperidol, which is more potent, may be given in doses ranging from .5 to 10 milligrams. As with the stimulant medications, it is impossible to predict how much medication a given child will require. Sometimes a very large, very active child may require a comparatively small dose, whereas a small and somewhat quieter child may require a larger dose. For this reason, as with stimulants, the physician will generally begin with a small dose, gradually increasing the amount until the problems seem to be well controlled. The parents should therefore expect that the doctor will frequently increase the dose at first, and they should not be upset because of this. To simplify the giving of medication, tablets of different sizes are generally used. The physician usually begins with the smallest dose tablet, to permit flexibility, and then substitutes larger tablets so that the child need not take a fistful of pills every day.

An important point about treatment with tranquilizers is that they are among the medications that sometimes require several weeks of administration before a maximum cumulative effect becomes apparent. Even after the correct dosage has been reached, full improvement may not be seen for several weeks.

Occasionally one finds a child in whom the medicines act long enough so that they can be given in only one dose a day. In such cases, medication is usually given every night, approximately 1 or 2 hours before the child's bedtime. The sleep effect of the medication appears approximately an hour after the medicine is given and wears off after 4 to 6 hours. (As mentioned, during the first few days or weeks the sleepiness will be more marked.) If the medicine is given 1 or 2 hours before bedtime it will assure a good night's sleep and will not make the child very groggy in the morning. Usually, however, the medicine does *not* appear to have a long-lasting effect and may have to be given two or three times a day.

Side effects

One very serious side effect produced by major tranquilizers consists of involuntary muscular movements usually of the lips, tongues, hands, and feet. The risk of this side effect, which is called tardive dyskinesia, increases with the dose and the time administered. If allowed to progress too far it is irreversible. When caught in its early phases, it usually is reversible. The possibility of this side effect does not mean that major tranquilizers should never be used. They should be used only when necessary and in as low doses and for as brief a time as possible. The decision to administer them should be made for each child individually, and the parent should remember that for some children they are absolutely necessary.

As mentioned in the general discussion of medication, most medications can produce allergies, and this is the case with the major tranquilizers. If allergies develop, they usually do so within the first few weeks or months of administration of a new medicine. Since developing allergies can sometimes be detected in the earlier stages by their effects on the blood count, some physicians obtain a blood count before the child starts the medication and at intervals thereafter. If a child has received the medication for a long time and has not developed an allergy, the risk of his developing one later is much smaller. For this reason, as time goes on, the physician will obtain blood tests less frequently or discontinue them altogether.

Another annoying, but not dangerous, side effect is the tendency of some of these medications to make children more susceptible to irritation by the sun. A few children who receive major tranquilizers and are exposed to the sun will develop an itchy rash. If this happens, the correct treatment is to have the child wear long-sleeved clothing and be out in the sun as little as possible.

A third annoying side effect, sometimes seen if children require comparatively large doses of these medications, involves some degree of muscular stiffness, shaking, and trembling. These symptoms are not serious and are routinely handled by giving another medicine that controls them.

Still other allergic symptoms can occur with these medications, as with any other, but they are rare. To be absolutely safe, a parent should notify the doctor of any unusual symptoms.

Although these side effects do occur in some children, they are infrequent. It is necessary to be aware of them, but it is not necessary to be very concerned about them.

Cyclic Antidepressants

A third group of medications that have proven useful in some ADD children consists of drugs commonly prescribed for the treatment of serious depressions in adults. Like the major tranquilizers, these drugs are used infrequently in ADD children, and they are absolutely nonhabit-forming. If given to an adult who is not depressed or to a child who is not hyperactive, they make the person irritable and/or anxious. They certainly do not make him high. A normal adult or nonhyperactive child would find the effects of these medications unpleasant and would not want to continue to take them. The antidepressants are not used routinely now for two reasons. First, they appear to be less effective than the stimulant medications. Fewer children respond. Among those who do, fewer ADD symptoms appear to improve. Even in those children for whom they work at first, tolerance to the medication often develops: the medication stops working, and increasing the dose does not restore its therapeutic effects. (The cyclic antidepressants may, however, be useful in the treatment of children who have both ADD and another psychiatric illness.) Second, as yet it is not known what effects these drugs would have if used in the treatment of ADD children over a period of years. Because the medical treatment of ADD children often requires that the medication be given daily for a number of years, physicians will need more experience with antidepressants given over a long period before prescribing them routinely.

As with the major tranquilizers, several kinds of antidepressants are available. The two most common are probably imipramine (Tofranil) and amitriptyline (Elavil).

Dosage

Most children who take antidepressants require between 30 and 200 milligrams of them a day. Since susceptibility to the medicines varies widely from child to child, the physician will generally begin with a low dose and gradually increase it over a period of several weeks, until either the child's symptoms improve or the side effects of the medicine become unpleasant. In some instances the usefulness of the medicine is immediately apparent; in others, the parent must be prepared to wait several weeks before it can be determined whether the medicine is helpful. There are slight differences among imipramine, amitriptyline, and the other medications, and sometimes a child may respond better to one than another. Since there is no way of predicting the child's responsiveness, the physician will often have to try several agents before reaching the best one.

As with the major tranquilizers, antidepressants sometimes produce some sleepiness the first few weeks they are administered. The sleepiness generally goes away with the passage of time. Generally, the physician will have to wait until the child has developed a tolerance to the sleepiness before increasing the dose of the medication.

Side effects

In addition to sleepiness, antidepressants sometimes produce other unpleasant nondangerous side effects, such as irritability, dry mouth, mild constipation, and mild dizziness. The side effects usually diminish after a while or can be controlled by lowering the dose slightly. Antidepressants rarely produce allergy, but as a precautionary measure periodic blood tests may be performed.

Other Medications

There are many other medications that sometimes prove effective when the above substances do not work. In rare instances a physician may have to try as many as six or eight, and the parents may have to wait several months before finding out if there is a medication that will benefit the child.

Recently, a few physicians have suggested the use of very large doses of vitamins in the treatment of children and adults with psychological difficulties, describing megavitamin therapy as a safe and effective treatment for several kinds of behavioral disorders. At present all one can say is that these claims are unsubstantiated. Nevertheless, the parent might believe that a trial use of large doses of vitamins would at least be natural and therefore safe. The difficulty is that although the vitamins are natural, doses of ten to a thousand times the normal daily requirement are not natural and may not be safe. Salt and water are natural, but someone who drinks many times the normal requirement of water in a day might well die of water intoxication. Although further information may show vitamin therapy to be effective and safe, there is now no evidence affirming that it is effective, and more evidence is needed to show that it is safe.

As can be seen from the above discussion, no medication used in the treatment of ADD children is ideal. Each medication has some disadvantages, usually minor. Researchers are constantly working to improve them, but in the meantime the medications available are usually effective (often dramatically so) and safe, and in the large majority of instances their advantages completely outweigh their disadvantages.

Aids to Administering Medication

Many parents to not realize it, but there are important psychological aspects to giving and taking medicine. This is usually overlooked because most medications are either for medical conditions or for obvious psychological ones. People take aspirin because of a headache, laxatives because of constipation, and tranquilizers because of anxiety. The hows and whys are straightforward. But in the administration of medicine to children for attention deficit disorder, several psychological principles play an important role. If treatment is to be maximally effective, these principles must be properly applied.

First, the child must have some understanding of why he is receiving medication. Second, he must be assured that taking medicine does not mean that his problems are terrible, such as being brain damaged or crazy. Third, it is useful to have him recognize and acknowledge problems in his own behavior *that he himself does not like*, so that he will not feel that medicine is being given to him simply so that other people can tolerate him more. If a child does not understand why he is receiving medication, if he does not feel that he has problems and that the medicine is helping him with these problems, he is likely to resist taking it, to forget taking it, or to discontinue taking it when he grows older but may still need it.

Usually an ADD child will recognize and acknowledge certain features of his experience and behavior that he does not like or that get him into trouble that he does not like. These may include such things as not being able to pay attention, having a hot temper, being "nervous" (restless), or being criticized by teachers or parents for forgetting things, not finishing work, or being out of the classroom seat all the time. He can honestly be told that the medicine will help him to complete his schoolwork, to pay attention, to hold his temper, to be less nervous, to remember things better, and to calm down. If he can accept the fact that the medicine is helping him, a large task has been accomplished. He will feel that something is being done for him rather than to him.

It is also important in giving medicine to children that they do not get the idea that because they have to take medicine they are somehow excused from assuming responsibility for their own behavior. ADD, like any other illness, does not negate free will. It may limit or modify someone's behavioral options, but it does not eliminate them. Children can and must feel that they share a responsibility for their behavior. They should not attribute all their actions to powers beyond their control. They should not be allowed to play the kind of "game" that Eric Berne, in his book Games People Play, calls wooden leg. In this psychological game, the person says the equivalent of "What can you expect of me? I couldn't do more. I've got a wooden leg." Children should be prevented from adopting the same attitude with regard to their ADD. They should not be allowed to imply: "I am a psychological cripple. I have ADD. All my actions are beyond my own control." For this reason, parents (and this applies to teachers and brothers and sisters as well) should not explain the ADD child's behavior on the basis of whether or not he's taken his medication. Parents should not say to him: "You are acting up. When did you have your medicine?" Putting things this way leads the child to believe that he has no control of himself, and it may put him in the position of having his "badness" explained by the absence of medicine and his "goodness" explained by its presence. If so, he can take no credit for controlling himself, and when he has not behaved in an appropriate way, he frequently can excuse himself because he hasn't taken his medication. If in talking to the ADD child, his parents, teachers, or brothers and sisters often associate his behavior with his medication schedule, he soon will learn how to play the game of "medicine wooden leg": "What can you expect of me? I have ADD and my medicine has worn off."

The importance of communicating to children their responsibility for their own behavior will become clearer in the section of this chapter entitled "Psychological Management."

Dietary Treatment

As I mentioned in Chapter 3, some physicians have suggested that ADD may be due to bodily reactions to normal food constituents. One possibility is that some children may be allergic to certain foods and the allergy may produce behavioral problems. A second, and different, claim has been made by a California physician, Dr. Ben Feingold (*Why Your Child is Hyperactive*, Random House, 1975), who believes that many children develop ADD as a reaction to artificial colorings, flavorings, some preservatives (which may be present in processed foods) and salicylates (a chemical related to aspirin) that are found naturally in some fruits and vegetables. A diet that eliminates these chemicals is called a food-additive-free or Feingold diet. The idea that food additives might cause ADD is particularly appealing to those people who believe that food additives are "unnatural" (and therefore probably harmful), and treatment with a special, healthful diet seems preferable to treatment with drugs. When children are put on these special diets without any attempt to disguise the treatment, some children do seem to show significant change in behavior. This is probably due to the change in the family's attitude about that child (which usually means more time spent with that child) and hopeful expectations in the minds of the child and his family. However, all the carefully conducted, controlled studies—in which the family does not know whether or not the child is on the additive-free diet—have shown that one type of additives (the artificial food colorings) does not produce significant hyperactivity (though it may produce some minor changes in attention in some children). Because there is still some room to hope that the food-additive-free diet may help *some* children, there would be no harm in families' trying this special diet as long as they pay attention to good nutrition and remain particularly alert to the need for vitamin C. (The Feingold diet limits the intake of several popular vitamin-C-containing fruits.) So far, however, I remain pessimistic about any relationship between food additives and ADD.

The subject of food allergies remains controversial. Some physicians believe that food allergies are frequently the cause of behavioral problems, while many others either doubt the existence of food allergies or think they occur infrequently and usually only in infants and toddlers. Doctors argue about this issue because there are no laboratory tests that can diagnose whether a food allergy exists. Therefore, the diagnosis must be made on the basis of clinical judgment—which means there is room for disagreement. Most physicians agree that the only certain way to diagnose food allergies is through an elimination diet. This usually involves removing all but the most basic, simple foods from the child's diet and then gradually, one at a time, adding foods back and observing the child's reaction. This is a tedious and time-consuming process that requires much patience on the part of both child and parent. For that reason, there has to be fairly good evidence that allergy may be a problem before most physicians are willing to try the elimination diet. It is my impression, as mentioned in Chapter 3, that the symptoms of food allergy are really different from the symptoms of true ADD. An occasional ADD child *may* show improvement if he is found to be allergic to certain foods and is placed on a diet that does not contain them. If parents think that food allergies may be causing problems for their child, it is probably a good idea for them to seek a physician's help in identifying possible allergies and then placing the child on a special diet that does not include the targeted foods. Although some pediatricians will investigate a child's possible food allergies, many would prefer that the child be seen by a pediatric allergist. It is important for parents to realize, however, that at present there is little evidence that food allergies play any substantial role in the behavior problems associated with hyperactivity.

Coffee

A few years ago someone proposed that ADD might be less common in South American countries—which may or may not be true—because children there drank coffee. Because coffee contains caffeine, a recognized stimulant of the brain, and because stimulants seem to help ADD, it was inferred that caffeine might be useful in treating ADD. A few studies have been conducted and they seem to indicate that caffeine, by itself, is *not* useful in treating ADD. When caffeine is combined with stimulant drug treatment, the overall response is better than with stimulant drugs alone, but the same good response can be obtained simply by increasing the amount of the stimulant drug. Because caffeine is less effective than the stimulant medication and has a variety of side effects that are considered undesirable, coffee does not have a useful place in the treatment of the ADD child.

PSYCHOLOGICAL MANAGEMENT

Most ADD children can benefit from medication and all of them can benefit from understanding and correct handling. ADD children have special problems but like all other children they may have "unspecial" ones as well. Difficulties, misunderstandings, friction between parent and child will cause trouble for any child. They may cause more trouble for the ADD child. This book focuses on the particular psychological problems the ADD child is likely to develop because of his difficulties in the areas of attention, impulsivity, and hyperactivity.

Understanding the Problem

The first part of this book has been devoted to a description of the typical problems of the ADD child and why he has these problems. It is very difficult to understand that a child who is attention-demanding, contrary, and short-tempered may be having a physical problem. Intuitively, one believes that he is having a psychological problem. As has been said, he does have psychological problems but they are physically caused.

If this is so, how should the parent handle the problems? It seems that if a problem is psychological the child is responsible for his behavior. If he is good he should be praised and if he is bad he should be punished. Similarly, if the problem is physical, the child is not responsible for his behavior. If that is so, he should not be rewarded for being good or punished for being bad. Neither of the above beliefs is true. Temperament may influence behavior but it is not the only factor that determines behavior. Temperament may make it easier or harder for a child to control himself. It may make it easier for him to learn to respond to discipline. But how the parents feel about the child and how they treat him can have appreciable effects.

During the past few years psychiatrists and psychologists have found that patients whose severe psychological problems are physically caused can be benefited markedly by psychological treatment. Mongolism, a severe form of retardation, is physically caused, but certain techniques of training can teach children with this disorder more effectively. Psychosis, severe psychological disturbances in adults, may produce childlike, withdrawn, or destructive behavior. These patients, whose symptoms are worse than those of any ADD child, can in many cases be helped by certain techniques. These techniques are based on three principles: (1) making the patients responsible for their behavior; (2) rewarding them for good behavior; (3) punishing them (in a special way) for bad behavior.

Similarly, the ADD child does better when he is held accountable and made responsible for his behavior. He should not be allowed to say, either in so many words or indirectly, "I'm hyperactive—I'm a mental cripple—I'm not responsible for what I do." He should be treated as responsible, and if necessary he should be told something to this effect: "You do have problems that may sometimes make it hard for you to control yourself. But the same thing is true for everybody. Everyone does some things more easily than others and does other things with more difficulty. You can learn to [count to ten, hold your temper, not tease your sister] and I expect you to." As with all my suggestions, of course, the parents should change the words to suit themselves and their children.

The child should not be held to be either irresponsible or blameworthy and should be treated as someone who has a greater tendency than average to do certain things. On the other hand, the parents should realize that for most ADD children no method of child rearing will eliminate certain tendencies. The child will tend to be more attention-seeking and forgetful, and will seem absentminded and willful. In most instances he is not doing these things to annoy. He would do them no matter how he had been raised. This distinction between symptoms that can be benefited by both rearing and medicine and those that can be alleviated only by medicine is important to remember. It will prevent the parent from trying to use psychological methods to change things that cannot be changed (or at best changed very little) in this way. Although psychologically unchangeable symptoms vary from child to child, they usually include the following: short attention span, distractibility, moodiness, lack of stick-to-itiveness, school underachievement, and immaturity. They *may* include bed-wetting, soiling, and some antisocial behaviors such as stealing. Again remember that although psychological techniques may not completely eliminate these problems in the child, they may help the child. For example, the child may continue to have tantrums, but he can be taught what to do when he has them. This will be discussed later.

In summary, there are three things the parent must remember. One, the child does have difficulties in doing and not doing certain things. Two, he will learn best how to compensate for his problems if he is treated as a responsible person who can gradually learn to control himself and his behavior. Three, the degree to which his problems can be helped by particular child-rearing techniques varies. It is much easier to teach him how to control his temper or how take responsibility for his chores than to teach him to have a longer attention span or to be less distractible. The first kind of problem (e.g., temper, chores) will be helped by both medicine and discipline. The second kind of problem (e.g., short attention span) for the most part can be helped only by medicine.

Basic Procedures

The main problem of the ADD child at home involves discipline. In discussing the basic procedures that will help the child to function effectively in his home environment, I will first indicate how the parents can establish constructive rules for the child. The second section will describe the rewards and punishments most likely to ensure that the child will adhere to these rules.

Establishing rules

Considerable evidence exists that certain ways of handling ADD children are more effective than others. It has been found that a firm, consistent, explicit, predictable home environment is the best. I will elaborate the special meaning that these terms have with respect to disciplining the ADD child. *Firm* means that rules and/or expectations for the child always have the same consequences. If he breaks a particular rule, he is always punished and always in the same way. If he does what he is asked, he always obtains acknowledgement and/or praise. *Consistent* means that the rules themselves do not change from day to day. If he is supposed to clean up his room before going out to play he is never allowed to leave his room until it has been cleaned up. *Explicit* means clearly defined and clearly understood by all parties. For example, cleaned up could mean that clothes have been hung in the closet, or that the bed has been made, or that toys have been returned to a shelf, or that the room has been vacuumed and dusted, or any combination of these things. For the cleaning-up rule, the definition of cleaning up must be explicit enough so that the child and the parents understand the rule the same way. *Predictable* means that laws are made before, not after the crime.

Obviously, all the parental expectations for the child cannot be stated beforehand. Parents never consider telling the toddler not to put nail polish on the rug and never think of telling him not to put a toy car in his ear. Some things can be dealt with only after they happen. In general, however, for most daily activities, rules can and should be made and then enforced. The child must wash himself, brush his teeth, do his around-the-house chores and homework every day; rules concerning these routine functions should be established. Punishment should follow any violation of the rules, but should not be employed if the rules have not been agreed on beforehand. Analogous consistent and predictable rules for adults exist in the speed limits for driving. It is easier to abide by a specific speed limit, say 55 mph, than adhere to the vague limit, "reasonable and proper," that was formerly designated in some Western states. In the case of the vague speed limit one does not know how fast he can go if it is twilight and a light rain is falling. Someone who is fearful may drive 35 mph. Someone who is more adventurous and drives at 40 mph may rightly be upset when she gets a ticket.

The above suggestions may impress parents as harsh and possibly cruel. They may also seem to contradict various benign permissive doctrines that advocate allowing children to "do their own thing," and allow opportunities for parents and children to talk things over. Let me correct some common misconceptions. First, firmness is not the same as harshness. Harshness is excessively severe or brutal rule enforcement. It is harsh to imprison someone for life for driving too fast. It is firm to fine him every time he does so. Second, children need structure. They need established rules, expectations, and values by which to live. Such structure does not mean the absence of freedom.

All people living in society have to follow certain rules and expectations if that society is to function effectively. Adults must not steal, drive when drunk, or embezzle. They must not urinate in public. Behaving in accordance with such rules also benefits the individual. First, and obviously, it keeps him out of trouble. But it also helps some individuals directly. Someone who has only poorly learned to control his impulses must consume a large part of his energy in simply controlling himself. The reformed alcoholic or drug addict must expend a great deal of effort in preventing himself from backsliding. The person who has learned to control himself readily has energies that he can utilize profitably elsewhere.

Note that this is not contrary to self-expression or creativity. The person who can handle his energies can create. The person who cannot channel his energies may be brilliant but will not be productive (consider the old saw that genius is 1 percent inspiration and 99 percent perspiration). Firm, consistent rules for behavior have nothing at all to do with the child's self-expression, nor understanding between parent and child. I have been talking about rules for behavior, not rules for thoughts and feelings. Thoughts and feelings are very different from behavior. They cannot be regulated and the parent should not attempt to regulate them. As discussed later, parents should help their children acknowledge and express their feelings. But both the parent and the child should always discriminate between feelings and behavior. For example, the parents of an ADD child should allow him to express his jealous feelings toward his newborn sister, but he should not be allowed to hit her. Feeling jealous and hitting because of jealousy should be recognized as being as different as night and day.

Finally, the setting of firm rules need not interfere with helpful discussions between the parents and the child. As the child becomes older such discussions certainly should be a part of family life, but even when he is younger they may be helpful. The child may, for example, suggest ways of getting his tasks done in a way that he likes better and that does not compromise the family. This is perfectly acceptable and in fact should be encouraged. But talking things over should not prevent rules from being formulated. It may influence how they are decided on and it may modify their exact terms but it should not interfere with their being established explicitly and consistently.

What evidence is there that the kind of structure discussed here is useful? Very interesting information comes from a study done in the middle thirties with severely hyperactive children. The behavior of these children was so uncontrollable at home that they had to be placed in a hospital for children with this serious behavior problem. The physicians had no previous experience with such children and tried various techniques to see which would be most effective. They began by assuming that the problems of the children were the result of excessive emotional stress and strain, and they treated them with a great deal of tolerance. This technique produced a brief period of improvement, which was soon followed by a recurrence of the same behavioral problems. Next, since the children had never received psychotherapy, they were treated in individual psychotherapy. This approach, too, proved unsuccessful. Finally, the doctors decided to create an environment that was "constructive," "restrictive," and "tolerant." The rules were not lax, and definite compliance to them was expected of the children. Children were isolated but not criticized for impulsive behavior (I will discuss this isolation later), and after they had calmed down they were helped to express themselves. The last technique clearly produced the greatest benefit, and many children could be discharged from the hospital to their homes. Unfortunately, those children who returned to homes where the parents could not be firm often again became disturbed and had to return to the hospital. It is important to emphasize that not all children were benefited by this (or any other) technique, but it was the technique that worked best.

This and similar studies give us reason to believe that environments structured in such ways can help ADD children. There is also reason to believe that they are most effective if begun early in life and that they are relatively ineffective (perhaps useless) if begun very late in childhood. The techniques to be discussed may help the preschool or young school-age child a great deal. They may be totally ineffective with an ADD child who is approaching adolescence.

What the specific rules should be in a particular family depends on parental preference and the age of the child. Parents could theoretically make any rules and teach young children to abide by them. (Different cultures have vastly different rules and standards for child behavior, and each culture succeeds in making a "standard product," a child well adapted to living in that culture.) As the child grows older, the parents' latitude decreases. The young child is for the most part only aware of how his own family does things. The older child is very much aware of how other children and their families do things, and will tend to rebel if his parents' standards appear different. A mother may keep her two-year-old boy in long curls and he will not protest. But it would be foolish of her to try to give her fourteen year old a prep-school-style haircut if his friends look like the latest pop idol. The earlier that rules and values are taught to a child the more likely he will be to maintain them later, even in the face of different standards outside the family.

The techniques to be discussed work best on younger children, say, up to the age of ten or eleven. These methods, which require that the child still be dependent on and controlled by his parents, are not for teen-agers—they need a different psychological approach.

With younger children, the first task for parents is to decide, concretely and specifically, what behaviors of the child require limitations or change. It is important to be concrete and specific so that the rules can be stated clearly and explicitly. Let me give some examples of vague, meaningless rules and how they can be clarified.

A. "He should clean his room." As I have indicated, this rule is highly ambiguous. If by "cleaning the room" the parent means put everything away and the child understands make your bed, he can feel wronged if he makes his bed, leaves, and is criticized. Furthermore, there is room for endless debate. The child cleaned the room by his standards but did not clean it by his mother's. We will return to this particular topic later in the subsection entitled "Chores."

B. "He should have better table manners." This might mean: he should eat with his fork instead of his fingers; he should put a napkin on his lap; he should say "please"; he should not use a boardinghouse reach, etc.

C. "He should treat his little sister better." This could mean: he should not hit her; he should allow her to play with his toys; he should not retaliate if she hits him, etc.

D. "He should be neater." This might mean: he should tie his shoelaces; button his shirt; wash his face; brush his teeth.

Not only does the child not know what his parents mean if they are not specific—and he can and will argue with them in the best legalistic fashion about what they might have meant—but also parents will have a much harder time determining whether progress has really taken place.

The second task of the parents is to establish a hierarchy of importance of rules. They must decide what is essential, what is important, what would be nice, and what is trivial. The parents must decide what are five-star rules and what are one-star rules. They must fit the punishment to the crime; they must distinguish between felonies and misdemeanors. They must not, so to speak, punish illegal parking with life imprisonment and punish murder with a warning. For example, parents have been known to use a talk as punishment for the setting of a serious fire, and a severe spanking as punishment for poor homework. The usefulness of establishing five- and one-star rules is that it helps parents to concentrate on the more important areas first and gives the child some breathing room. After the most essential problems have been brought under control, the parents can move to the next category.

Another task for the parents is to predecide that both mother and father will abide by the prescribed course of action. This policy is not always easy to carry out. Frequently, each parent has devised his or her own (usually not too successful) technique for dealing with the child, and unfortunately each often believes that that technique is right and the child's problems are the result of the other's mismanagement. If such a family atmosphere exists, it conflicts with the consistent united front that is an absolute requirement for helping the ADD child learn to control his behavior. It is not necessary for the parents to agree completely with each other—they simply must act in common. If the parents are incapable of resolving their differences and agreeing on rules and standards for their ADD child's behavior, they may benefit from psychological assistance. A psychiatrist, social worker, or psychologist may enable them to thrash out their differences and determine the set of rules, and the relative importance of the various rules, necessary for their ADD child.

Rewards and punishments

In addition to establishing sound rules to help the child, the parents must predecide a plan of rewards and punishments. The rewards and punishments should be seen as such by the child and not only by the parents. The words reward and punishment have an unfortunate meaning to some people. Reward seems to suggest bribery and punishment seems to suggest brutality. All that is meant by reward is something the child likes, particularly attention, praise, or a small special privilege. Certain privileges, toys, and so forth can be useful under special conditions, which will be discussed later.

Similarly, punishment simply means something the child does not like. It does not mean beating, or depriving of privileges for a long time. Generally, with younger children, a most effective and nonhurtful punishment is sending the child to his room until he stops behaving in an undesirable way (e.g., having a tantrum) or finishes a required task (e.g., getting dressed). It is more effective to say, "Go to your room, please, and come back to breakfast when your shoes are tied and your face is washed," than it is to yell at the child and/or beat him.

There are two more important principles of reward and punishment. First, to be most useful, a reward or punishment should be immediate. Any delay decreases effectiveness. When a child does what you want him to, praise him on the spot. If he does what he has been told not to do, punish him at once. Do not offer distant presents ("any toy you want two weeks from now") or threaten punishment ("Daddy will spank you when he gets home"). Second, the one-time rule should be adopted. The parents should learn the habit of saying do or don't only *once* before rewarding or punishing. If they do not apply this rule, if they give first, second, third, and tenth warnings before acting, their children will learn to commit ten violations before worrying. In the meantime the parents will have developed a sore throat and built up a good head of angry steam. In some cases, the child may have been anxiously pushing his parent to take a stand. Surprisingly, most children are relieved when the parent finally acts. A good deal of friction can be avoided by the use of this one-time rule.

In the past forty years, psychologists have learned a great deal about reward and punishment from animal experimentation. Researchers have discovered extremely simple and effective techniques that can be used to teach lower animals, such as pigeons and rats, to perform very complicated tasks. For example, it is fairly easy to teach a rat to push a bar for food when a certain colored light is on and to push another bar to avoid receiving a shock when another light is on. Using these techniques, one can teach a rat to push a bar very slowly for food under one set of conditions and very rapidly under another set.

In the past twenty-five years or so, psychologists have found that such techniques are sometimes helpful in teaching and controlling the behavior of human beings whose psychological difficulties are so great that previously they seemed unreachable by any known technique—for example, profoundly retarded children and adults, children of normal intelligence who are unable to talk, and seriously disturbed adult psychiatric patients. In more recent years a number of psychologists have tried applying these operant techniques to children with behavioral problems. The operant techniques—or operant conditioning—are no more than refined sets of rewards and punishments, and the work of the psychologists can be translated into recommendations that can be very helpful to parents of ADD children.

The exact rules and laws of operant conditioning as they are used in the laboratory are somewhat complicated, but the basic principle that parents can use is exceedingly simple. It is that *acts are influenced by their consequences.* That is, what happens after an animal or child does something greatly influences, either positively or negatively, the likelihood of his doing the same thing again. For the parents, this means that how they act when their child does or says something will either increase or decrease the probability that the child will behave that way again.

This principle is most easy to illustrate in the use of operant conditioning with animals. In a typical experiment a hungry rat is placed in a simple cage with a bar in it. In the course of his explorations the rat eventually leans on the bar. When he does so a pellet of food is released automatically into the feeding dish. If one observes the rat through a one-way screen one sees that the rat may not return to the bar for a while. Eventually, perhaps by accident, he will depress the bar again, and again will be rewarded by food. As one continues to watch the rat, one finds that he eventually seems to get the idea. After a day or two of training in such a cage the hungry rat will immediately go to the bar and press it. Notice that I use the phrase *get the idea*. Obviously there is no information about the consciousness of rats, and the phrase may be somewhat misleading, but in humans such behavior can be learned without awareness: some experiments seem to indicate the subjects may learn to change some kinds of behavior with no awareness whatsoever of the sequence that produces the change. That is, people may develop habits that produce certain consequences for them without being aware of any relationship between the habits, the acts based on those habits, and the consequences of those acts.

To illustrate the principle in animal experimentation again, I will describe a typical demonstration in an elementary psychology course. A hungry pigeon is placed in a cage. Standing outside the cage and observing the pigeon through a one-way screen is the experimenter. In his hand he holds a switch that he can use to cause a click to be made in the box and a kernel of corn delivered to the pigeon in a feeding dish. The experimenter may choose to make the pigeon perform any behavior pigeons are capable of. In one instance it was decided to make the pigeon rotate counterclockwise, spinning like a ballerina. In order to accomplish this, the experimenter waited until the pigeon in his normal wanderings had turned slightly to the left. After the pigeon had done so, the experimenter pressed the switch and the pigeon received a kernel of corn. In the next 20 or 30 seconds the pigeon again turned to the left, and the experimenter delivered another kernel of corn. In the following few minutes the pigeon began to rotate slowly toward his left. After he had done so for a while the experimenter again delivered a kernel of corn. During the next 5 or 10 minutes the pigeon began to turn continuously in a circle. The experimenter would wait until the pigeon was turning rapidly and then, and only then, deliver the food. Thereafter, when the pigeon turned slowly he received no food and when he turned rapidly he received the food. At the end of the half hour the class was astonished to see a pigeon rotating like a whirling dervish. This experiment illustrates the complex tasks that can be taught even to lower animals. More complex behavior can be taught to humans, and (as cannot be illustrated by animal experiments) such learning can apparently occur without the person's awareness of it as well as with his being conscious of it.

Before examining the question of what relevance these experiments have for people, let me digress for just a moment and define two, and only two, terms from operant conditioning therapy. The first term is operant, and the second is reinforcement. An operant is any voluntary act an animal or human being is capable of performing. It includes the rat's bar-pressing and the pigeon's circling. In fact, it includes most behavior. In children it might even include talking, attention-getting, having tantrums, waking up in the middle of the night, lying, stealing, crying, fire-setting, writing poems, or philosophizing—in short, almost anything. Reinforcement is synonymous with the word reward. In the animal experiments discussed, reinforcement was food. Food is rewarding or reinforcing to a hungry animal.

What is reinforcing to children? That depends on their state. To the rat who has eaten his fill, food is no longer reinforcing, and he will not depress a bar to obtain it. In working with very disturbed psychiatric patients, therapists have occasionally used food as a reinforcer; such a procedure can sometimes be effective if the patients are kept somewhat hungry. Similarly, for a thirsty child, water can be reinforcing; for a hungry child, food can be reinforcing. However, most of the child's acts are influenced by parental behavior that is quite different from simple satisfaction of hunger or thirst. For an individual child, reinforcing behavior varies, *but certain parental acts and behaviors are reinforcing to almost all children.* The most important, as I have suggested, are parental affection and parental attention. Parental attention is probably the single most common reinforcer in a child's daily life. It is important not only because of the frequency with which it is focused on the child, but also because it is reinforcing no matter what elicits it. Some kinds of punishment, therefore, are more rewarding to a child than ignoring him. Expressing disapproval of a child's most recent misdeed is giving him attention. Thus, paradoxically, the likelihood that a child will repeat a misdeed may be increased when the parent discusses the misdeed with the child at too great a length.

What about more severe punishment? The reinforcers I have discussed are referred to by psychologists as positive reinforcers. What the layperson refers to as punishment, the psychologist calls negative reinforcement. Certain general principles have been learned about the effects and effectiveness of negative reinforcement.

To begin with, negative reinforcement *generally* reduces the likelihood of the repetition of the act that preceded it. Thus, as generations of parents have learned, with most children most of the time a good spanking is a pretty effective way of preventing a child from doing again what he just did that the parents didn't like. The rat who received a powerful electric shock after pressing the bar will refrain from doing so in the future or, at least, in the very near future. Psychologists have also learned some less obvious things about punishment. If it is very severe (e.g., a very painful electric shock, which is almost enough to paralyze the animal), the animal is likely *never* to repeat the act again, but punishments of this nature are also likely to be accompanied by side effects that change the animal in a number of undesirable ways. Animals that receive such powerful punishment are apt to become erratic and often show disturbed (neurotic) behavior in other areas. In experiments in which electric shocks have been used to teach dogs to avoid things, the dogs have become vicious, excited, withdrawn, or very fearful. In other words, punishment that is effective enough to prevent offensive behavior permanently may produce more disturbing behavior than what it prevented.

If, then, some punishment focuses attention on the child and therefore reinforces poor behavior, and if severe punishment is likely to produce bad side effects, the question arises as to whether any forms of punishment can be reasonably effective. Although psychologists disagree, it seems that there are lesser degrees of punishment that can suppress behavior but only temporarily. That is, shocks that will not make the animal neurotic are not likely to be effective for very long. The relevance of this for children should be fairly obvious. Humane parents use only moderate punishment and, in ADD children, who are often not particularly responsive to punishment, the effects of punishment should not be expected to be long-lasting. And in fact they rarely are.

Positive reinforcement, on the other hand, may not be permanent either, but with certain modifications may be extremely long-lasting. Its virtue is that once the child is started on the right track he is likely to receive reinforcement from people outside the family. The child who is taught to be reasonably polite, moderately obedient, and reasonably nonaggressive will be reinforced by favorable attention from others, by making friends and succeeding.

One other feature of positive reinforcement increases the possibility that it may have very long-lasting effects and it can also be illustrated by animal experimentation. When a rat is trained to push a bar, he receives food on every bar press. If one stops delivering a pellet each time the rat presses the bar, after a while the rat pushes less and less frequently and eventually stops. However, with a simple modification of the experiment, the rat can be made to work a much longer time for fewer pellets. Let us suppose we arrange the machine so that at first the rat receives a pellet only on every second bar push. Then after a while we arrange it so that he receives a pellet on every third, and every fourth, and so on. Now suppose we tinker around with the machinery (and this is very simple) so that the rat is playing a slot machine, that is, he receives a pellet, *on the average*, on every 20th or 50th or 100th bar press. Sometimes he receives three pellets in a row. Sometimes he may have to press the bar 200 times before receiving a pellet. After a rat has been exposed to this payoff system he is very resistant to losing his habit. Again the relevance of this to children should be obvious. One begins by reinforcing the child every time he performs a desired behavior. After a while one changes the payoff and gradually reinforces him less for the same behavior. Like the rat in whom reinforcement has been tapered off in the same way, the child is now likely to persist in this behavior even without a constant payoff.

Having criticized punishment (and not for humane grounds but for practical grounds), I must back down a little and point out that it does have some effectiveness and that it can be important in situations that are dangerous or life-threatening. The two year old rushing out into the street (to possible death) should be punished fairly severely and immediately. This will decrease the likelihood of his doing it again in the near future. One is more likely to keep him out of the street, however, if he is positively reinforced for doing things that prevent his going there (e.g., staying on the lawn or playing in the backyard). Punishment is a good temporary technique but it is ineffective in the long run in most ADD children.

One point I've touched on but must emphasize is the question of when reinforcement should occur. One word will suffice: *immediately*. In the experiments with animals, the success of the technique depends on the animal's receiving the reinforcement the moment after the act—the operant—is performed. A delay of one second decreases its effectiveness a little, a delay of five seconds reduces it considerably, a delay of a minute makes it useless. Children apparently can tolerate longer delays but the same principle applies to them. Positive reinforcement (or reward) and negative reinforcement (or punishment) are much more effective if they are received immediately. If a child does what the parent wants him to do, he should receive praise for that act immediately. If he does something that requires punishment, he should be punished immediately. It is ineffective and a waste of time to promise to reward the child in two weeks if he obtains good grades now or to delay necessary punishment until Daddy comes home. Such reinforcements *may* work at best temporarily (two weeks, or the rest of the day) but will have no long-lasting effect.

From this discussion the question emerges of how these techniques should be applied practically to children. They may be used informally and formally. Clearly, an important principle of their informal application is that children should be positively reinforced, immediately, when they do what their parents want. Once the child knows what his parents' desires are (e.g., putting his shoes away, eating with a fork, saying "please"), he should be reinforced by his parents in a specific way whenever he performs these acts. By specific I mean that the parents should comment on the desired behavior in believable and pertinent terms. If he is asked to put his shoes away and does so, the parent should not say, "You are a wonderful son"; he or she should say, "I am very pleased that you are learning to take care of your things like a grown-up boy," or words to that effect. Children, like adults, recognize overgeneral praise as false. The child should know what he is receiving praise for.

Theoretically, the corresponding principle to be applied when children behave undesirably would require that the children be ignored, but how can the parent ignore undesirable behavior? If the child is acting like a clown, it is easy. If he is pummeling his three-year-old sister or destroying the house, ignoring him is dangerous and/or expensive. If he is engaging in harmless attention-seeking behavior, ignoring is easy. If he is engaged in behavior that is destructive or harmful, ignoring should be combined with the isolation-room technique.

The usefulness of the isolation room becomes apparent when one considers what ordinarily happens when a child misbehaves. For example, if the child punches his sister, the parent is apt to ask at least, "Why did you do that?" Thus, the child receives attention for misbehaving. In accordance with the principles discussed, attention is likely to increase the probability that the child will do the same thing again. In other words, the parents' normal discussion with the child is likely to result in greater future misbehavior. With the isolation-room technique, the child is informed beforehand that whenever he misbehaves he will be sent to his room. Then when he actually does misbehave he is simply told that he is going to his room and that he will be allowed to come out as soon as he regains control of himself. If he goes willingly, that is fine. If he has to be carried, that may not be fine but it is effective. If he tries to leave his room, then a screen-door latch should be placed on the outside and locked.* When the child quiets down—or, in the case of the older child, when he announces that he has quieted down and comes out himself—then, and only then, does

---

*Parents should *never* leave the house while the child is locked in the room, because of the always present (even though remote) possibility of fire or similar emergency.

the parent sit down with the child and discuss what was bothering him before. With this technique the child receives attention for being in control of himself, not for being out of control. After a child has had considerable experience with this procedure, he often learns to go to his room when he has become upset and to come out when he is no longer upset. If the child has to be kept in the room, the parents should not let him out until he is able to be in control of himself—that is, until his tantrum has stopped or his anger outburst is under control. This technique has been used effectively with very disturbed hospitalized psychiatric patients as well as with hyperactive children. It is an especially effective technique with young (under the age of nine or ten) ADD children.

The second way in which reinforcement therapy can be applied, the more formal way, cannot be used with the youngest ADD children, but is effective with children beyond, say, the age of six. With this method the parent and the child decide what tasks the parents would like the child to perform. These may be tasks that occur every day or once a week. They may, for example, include making his bed, putting his clothes in the hamper, or taking out the trash. A weekly chart is kept and the parent and the child predecide how many tokens—for example, poker chips—the child will receive for performing as agreed. Whenever the child does do the work, he promptly receives the predecided number of poker chips. The child is allowed to accumulate the credits he earns for desirable behavior and can exchange them later for objects or for privileges he regards as desirable. In other words, he earns tokens and spends them for the movies, going out to play, watching TV, or, if the parents choose, even for money. In any event, the rate of exchange should also be decided on beforehand. This technique will be further described in the subsection entitled "Chores."

Contingency contracting

Contingency contracting is a behavioral technique more suited for use with older children. The notion is very simple. Parents and children discuss what each desires from the other in very specific terms. In one example, a child's obligation might be cleaning up his room each morning, and the reward from the parent might be permission to watch television for an agreed-on time. The difference from the behavior modification techniques already described is that the parent and child engage in collective bargaining—comparable to that between unions and management. The child plays an active role in establishing the bargain and the standards by which his performance will be judged. In this instance it might include such items as bed made, clothes removed from floor and placed in hamper, towels hung up in bathroom, etc. Likewise, the parents specify what they will do or permit when the contract is fully or partially fulfilled. Such a contract is typically made in writing, with each party clearly stating his obligations and the obligations of the other party, and is signed by the child and each of the parents. It is called a contingency contract because the arrangement is, "If you do this, I will do that, and if I do that, you will do this." Each person's behavior is contingent—that is, dependent—on that of the other party to the contract. This kind of explicit bargaining has been used widely in dealing with hospitalized mental patients and is used by some therapists who practice behavioral family therapy. It has a ring of reasonableness about it, but its effectiveness has yet to be proven scientifically.

The above techniques may seem very mechanical to the parent who has diligently read books on child guidance and child rearing. Most of these books stress that children misbehave because of deep-seated underlying problems, or lack of understanding of their own feelings. A valuable principle that has been provided by the operant therapists is that although these statements can be true, children are also mightily influenced by the consequences of their acts. Love is not enough. Understanding is not enough. If a child is to learn to behave desirably, his parents must become aware of what their own reactions are in response to his various kinds of acts.

A child may behave well without understanding or he may misbehave with full insight into what he is doing. The child may accurately describe himself as angry when he hits his baby sister. This is an interesting instance of the child's ability to comment on his own behavior. It is not helpful to his baby sister. For the child to be helped, and for the family to be helped, the child must learn to control his own behavior. If the child is to feel good about himself he may also have to learn about his own feelings. Helping the child understand himself and deal with his feelings will be discussed in the next section.

Helpful General Principles and Techniques

The general question of how parents should treat their children, of how they should relate to them in order to produce the healthiest possible psychological environment, has been the subject of numerous books. They carry a wealth of helpful advice for parents of all kinds of children, and no effort can be made here to review every approach that psychologists have found useful. However, certain general principles and techniques that are of special benefit to ADD children as well as to children with no problems will be discussed briefly. When added to the previous discussion of basic procedures, they provide a good picture of psychological approaches that can be particularly useful in managing the ADD child.

How to criticize

No one likes criticism and children are no exception. Everyone can tolerate criticism best when it is specific, not generalized. For example, the husband who arrives home from work and finds supper not ready could respond with either of these two statements: "You are a terrible wife and never get anything done," or, "I'm always starving after work and I'd really appreciate it if you could have dinner ready when I get home." The wife might not like either of the two statements but the second, being more specific and somewhat more understanding, is a lot easier to take. Similarly, an employer faced with a problem of chastising an employee who is late finishing a piece of work could select one of the following statements: "Jones, you are a lousy worker," or, "Jones, I'd appreciate it in the future if you'd be faster in getting me these reports."

Again, the employee may not like *any* criticism, but the second version, being specific, is easier to swallow.

The same principle applies to criticism of children. When, for example, the ADD child has just hit his baby sister for picking up his favorite toy, reducing her to a howling mass, the parent is likely to explode and say such things as: "Why must you be such a bad child?" "You're a terrible child and you're always making trouble!" "Can't you do anything right?" Reacting this way is understandable. Nevertheless, such an explosion is not helpful. If parents have thought about the problem areas in which improvement is wanted, they are in a far better position to criticize specifically. For example: "I told you not to hit your baby sister. That hurts her and makes me angry. Please go to your room." Other examples: "I do not like it when you eat with your hands—that is for small babies, not big children"; "Mommy gets upset when she asks you to clean up your room and you do not. Nobody likes to look at messy rooms. Please go back and clean it." In the examples given, the parent expresses anger—but about *specific acts*. It is perfectly all right and it is sensible for the parent to acknowledge feelings that a child knows are present. The child can see that the parent is angry. Denying what the child knows is not useful. But the parents must not allow their anger to take the form of criticizing the child as a whole. The parents must never call the child worthless or bad. When criticism is necessary, the parents should criticize the objectionable behavior and be as specific as possible.

How to praise

Similarly, praise should be specific. Affectionate attention should be provided when the child is behaving desirably. If the child is eating nicely, say, "You are eating in a very grown-up fashion and that pleases me." If his baby sister is teasing him and he has resisted the urge to slug her, say, "I am very pleased that you can hold your temper even when Susie is making a pest of herself."

It is not very helpful to say, "You are a wonderful child," or to tell your spouse, "Jimmy has been just marvelous today." In addition to being ineffective in helping the child achieve self-control, such comments are likely to strike him as phony. All of us react to such comprehensive praise as false. We all know we have our good and bad points and that anybody who calls us "wonderful" is either trying to butter us up or is stupid. Children have the same reaction. Consider the TV talk show in which an actor is introduced as a "wonderful personality." That turns most of us off. We recognize it for the hokum it is. Thus, when you do praise children, praise them for the specific things that they have done that they know are good. Do not enlarge. Children recognize and appreciate honesty.

Recognizing the child's feelings

The general principle here is that children, like adults, need to be understood, especially by someone important to them. Children have feelings. Recognizing those feelings and letting the child know that you recognize them often helps the child to feel better. It is extremely important, however, to realize that a parent can recognize a child's feelings and communicate that recognition without either criticizing or praising him. If the child is returning from his room, where he has been sent because of lack of control, the parent can help by saying something like "You must have felt that it is very difficult for a seven year old to always remember his table manners, and you must have been angry at Mommy for making you leave the table."

By recognizing and acknowledging feelings in a neutral way, the parent can make the child feel more comfortable.

Helping the child distinguish between feelings and actions

The major principle here is that feelings can and should be expressed, even if they are bad. A part of the same principle is that feelings and actions are not the same thing. Children, like adults, often have feelings that "they should not"; they are sometimes envious, jealous, angry, resentful. All children have these feelings. In certain circumstances everyone has them. Children often feel guilty about having such feelings. They have learned that one should not be envious, jealous, angry, or resentful. It is very helpful if the parents, as discussed in the previous section, acknowledge to themselves that the child has such feelings (when he does) and let the child know that they (the parents) know. The parents must help the child distinguish between feelings (which are acceptable) and actions (which are not). Actions—that is, behavior—can be changed and shaped; feelings cannot be changed so directly and should not be treated as if they could be. If the child sees that his parents recognize and tolerate his feelings, his anxiety about having them may be relieved. His relief alone may often release enough steam so that the child will not act on his bad feelings. The child will feel less guilty if he knows that bad thoughts do not mean that he is bad and worthless in his parents' eyes. Since in the past he has acted in ways that have been considered unacceptable, he is likely to regard having comparable thoughts as equally reprehensible. The parents should repeatedly communicate to the child, directly and indirectly, that any bad thoughts that he might have are not terrible so long as he does not act on them. He will sometimes feel very angry at his baby sister; he should express such anger and his parents should help him express such angry feelings. He should not hit his baby sister. Parents should help the child to understand the difference between thinking and doing.

The technique of labeling

One extremely important technique in helping the ADD child to recognize and do something about his behavioral problems is labeling. Before the child can even begin to attempt to control his own behavior, he must know when he is doing something that is troublesome to others or hurtful to himself. The catch is that many of these things are rather complicated. It is easy for the parent to tell the child, "When you lie down on the floor, scream, and pound your heels, that is a tantrum," and "Mommy will not talk to you until the tantrum is over, and if you cannot make it stop quickly you will have to go to your room until it is over." A three year old can learn what a tantrum is. But some of the ADD child's trouble-producing behaviors are more complex than that.

For example, he may devise sophisticated techniques—and have a variety of them—for bugging his brother or sister. His father and mother cannot draw up a complete list of bugging behaviors. An enterprising, intelligent ADD child can find multiple ways of annoying others. In order to help the child identify and recognize such behaviors, the parents should choose a code word. The code words I use are bugging and teasing. Every time the ADD child bothers his brother or sister this way, the child is told, "You are teasing." After a few dozen repetitions— and parents will have many, many opportunities in the course of time— the child learns to recognize that a whole group of different things can be called teasing. It is no harder for the child to learn this than it is for him to learn that Great Danes, Dachshunds, and Chihuahuas are all dogs.

Once the child has learned what teasing is, the parents can expand the usefulness of the procedure by dealing with new occurrences in a different way. When Billy is pretending that he has lost his sister's doll, the parent can say, "Billy, what are you doing?" The intention now is to have him label his own behavior, which is a step toward taking more responsibility for it.

Other examples of common problems for which labeling is a useful technique are having trouble with attention or getting excited. Parents should actively look for and invent labels for the particular problems of their ADD child that may lend themselves to this procedure. With repetitive labeling of this sort, the parents of the ADD child can generally help him to identify what he is doing. Remember that this is not easy. In *Games People Play*, Eric Berne spends a lot of time making up clever names for neurotic behaviors of adults. The reason the clever names are useful is that even adults, without the handicaps of ADD, do not easily recognize the different ways they can be neurotic or just plain difficult. It is not surprising that an immature ten year old will have a hard time learning what is objectionable about his behavior.

Scientific investigation of the usefulness of teaching children to recognize their own troublesome behavior is in an early stage. Interestingly, Russian child psychologists have for some time been examining the ways in which language can help a child to control himself.

They feel that self-labeling is the first step in self-control, and that the sooner the child learns to label what he is doing, the sooner he can learn to control himself. Although definitive evidence is not yet available, my clinical experience has impressed me with the usefulness of labeling as an additional parental technique.

The Management of Common Problems of the ADD Child

The procedures, principles, and techniques described above refer to overall approaches to the ADD child. In addition, I have some special suggestions that may be of help in managing a few specific common problems of the ADD child.

Getting the child's attention

One of the ADD child's major problems is paying attention. And one of the major problems of the parent of an ADD child is getting the child's attention. If one wishes to communicate effectively with an ADD child, one must use some special techniques. For example, often the parent will give a command to or make a request of an ADD preschooler while the child's attention is elsewhere. In non-ADD children such a parental request may catch the child's attention. In the case of the ADD child, it usually does not. Even if the parent has the ADD child's attention, the child may not wish to hear what the parent has to say and may place his hands over his ears or turn his head away. The procedure that should be employed is as follows: the parent should take the ADD child's head (or shoulders) gently in his (or her) hands and give the child the message. Then, to be sure that the child has received the message, the parent should ask the child what he was told, not in a punitive way but with a neutral tone. If the child does not know, the parent should make the statement again. Physical contact seems to play an important role in gaining the child's attention. When the message is given with the parent's hands placed on the child's shoulders, the child seems to pay better attention than he does when not touched.

Although the instructions above have mentioned the preschooler, physical contact may still be useful with the older child as well. So is the procedure of asking the child what it was that he was told. Parents should remember that if they find themselves yelling in order to get the child's attention, something has gone wrong someplace.

Rigidity

A characteristic of some ADD children—although it can be seen in non-ADD children as well—is rigidity. Rigid children are upset when their activities are interrupted or their routines changed. For example, they may become furious if they are stopped from playing with their toys so that they can be taken on a visit to Grandma's. Or they may begin screaming if the order of putting on their clothes is varied. One three-year-old ADD child had a tantrum if the family drove to Grandma's house by a different route.

Rigidity sometimes disappears with age, but there are effective ways of dealing with it before that blessed time comes. The major principle is anticipation. Long before the break in routine occurs, the parent should repeatedly tell the child what is going to happen. For example, if the child is playing with his blocks and cars and the time to leave for Grandma's is two hours in the future, the parent should begin a countdown: "Billy, we will be visiting Grandma in two hours." Then, an hour later, "We will be leaving in one hour. It's time for you to put the trucks away." Next, "Billy, we are leaving for Grandma's in 15 minutes. It's time to put the blocks away, change your clothes, and put your shoes on." With older children, to avoid repeated nagging, egg timers can be invaluable. Even before the child can tell time, he can recognize when the pointer is approaching the "0" that will start the bell. Rather than giving countdowns every morning for getting dressed to go to school, one can substitute the timer.

Similarly, considerable grief can often be avoided by discussing long-term changes before they occur. Repeated anticipatory talks about such matters as furniture moving, new sleeping arrangements, and altered school programs can frequently soften the blow for the rigid child. These procedures, of course, do not change the child's rigidity, but they lessen its unpleasant impact.

Spiraling loss of control

A very frequent problem of ADD children, both as preschoolers and during the first few grades, is a spiraling loss of behavioral control. This refers to the child's becoming increasingly wild and behaving more and more immaturely once he is set off. For example, when guests come, the child may act in an attention-seeking manner, and as soon as he gets the attention he may react with foolish and noisy behavior that steadily worsens. After first telling the guests a story or showing them some of his models, he may begin to talk more loudly, to start running around, and in some instances to bounce off the walls. This may also happen in noisy or stimulating situations, such as at the supermarket or the circus.

How can this loss of control be handled? To begin with, it is helpful if parents learn to recognize the early symptoms of this behavioral breakdown. It is far easier to reverse such cycles shortly after they have started than when they are in full swing. When the parents recognize the symptoms of an impending behavior spiral, they should caution the child with a phrase that is always used when the child is excited—and here we see again the labeling technique in operation. Different parents use different phrases. Some parents will say, "You are getting too wild," while others might caution, "You are becoming overexcited." The important point is to label the same kind of behavior in the same way every time so that the child can learn what the parents mean by the special phrase. After the parent has identified the behavior, the child should be told to go to his own room and to remain there until he has calmed down. If necessary, he should be taken to his room. Once he has calmed down, the child should receive no punishment but in fact should receive praise for having gotten control of himself, and for now acting like a big boy. Then, in a nonaccusatory tone of voice, the parent should explain to the child what happened before and what caused the parent to label that behavior as wild or overexcited. In other words, parents should make sure that the child is praised (gets positive reinforcement) for acting quite grown-up, and that the child receives no extra attention—positive or negative—for being out of control.

Thus, the best thing to do about spiraling loss of control is to try to avoid it. To use a variation on an old cliché, parents should be ready with that invaluable ounce of prevention. They should learn to recognize the situations that trigger these spiraling reactions and either avoid them or remove the child from them as soon as possible.

Verbal tantrums

One of the kinds of loss of control seen in both younger and older ADD children is the verbal tantrum. Such behavior is probably more mature than breath-holding spells or down-on-the-floor kicking tantrums, but parents are not overjoyed at this kind of maturation. During the tantrum the child may talk (or yell) continuously, criticizing, blaming others, and denying responsibility. He may bring up not only trivial matters but honest-to goodness problems that exist in the family. The nonstop productions are limited only by his talkativeness and how his parents handle the problem. The natural reaction of most parents is to argue. The major advice that I have is that the parent should not argue at all. A mutual screaming match solves nothing. While the child is having the tantrum, he should be told that matters will be discussed when he quiets down. If he is unable to quiet down, he should be placed in a time-out room, and only *after* he quiets down should the parent talk with the child about the real problem. Parents who frequently find themselves yelling can interpret that as a warning sign that they are doing something wrong—not bad, just ineffective.

Chores

Although particular chores have been used as examples in the preceding sections, I am giving special attention to the entire subject of getting the child to do routine, age-appropriate chores because it is one of the most common causes of friction between the school-age ADD child and his parents. At first, nonperformance may be a result of forgetfulness and the child's inability to organize well. If the parents become angry and nag—and, except for a few saints, most become angry—the child may become increasingly stubborn and negative. This may lead to a snowballing of complaints by the parents and of goldbricking by the child.

The best way to make sure that chores are done is as follows. First, list all the chores you want the child to do. Second, arrange them in order of importance ("1" next to the most important task, "2" next to the second most important task, etc.). Then, write down one or two of the most important chores on a homemade calendar and place this calendar in a conspicuous place, say, on the refrigerator door. For example, if one chore is to set the table every other day (as sometimes happens when a brother or sister is also doing the same chore), the calendar should have the child's name listed on each day he is to perform it. If there are two chores involved, such as setting the table and clearing it, each should be listed separately on the day it is to be done (whether every day, on alternate days, or according to some other schedule).

Parents should avoid any disputes about what constitutes the chore by writing down its specific components. In setting the table, does one only have to place the silverware and dishes, or does one also have to bring the butter and milk from the refrigerator, and so forth? Assuming reasonably good parent-child relationships, many children will be compliant about chores if the requests are specific and structured enough.

If the child is resistant, the behavior modification principles I have mentioned should be employed. For example, parents could establish a rule saying that full payment of allowance will be made only if setting the table is done, without nagging, six times a week. With such a rule, if the chore is done only five times in a week, the child is docked in some mutually agreed-on way—such as receiving only five-sixths of his allowance.

After the most important chores are being done on a regular basis, the parents can move on to the next chore. Again, the calendar should be kept, and directions should be very clear and specific. Parents will avoid hassles if the rules are easy to understand and clear-cut. If they are not, the opportunity for legal arguments is much greater. And as all parents know, most children are born lawyers.

Having the child take responsibility for himself

All parents hope that eventually the child will take responsibility for monitoring his own behavior. The procedure discussed under "Chores" illustrates one way of establishing a habit of responsibility. Here I will describe another method of encouraging responsibility. The example deals with another recurrent problem of the ADD child—forgetting to bring his school assignments home, which means that he does not do his homework.

For this problem, I suggest that the child be given a small notebook in which he must write down *every day* after arriving home from school the work he actually accomplished at school and what was left undone in each subject that day. If homework assignments are given, he should write down those assignments while he is in school, in the same book. It is his responsibility to write this information down. At the end of the week, the parent should contact the child's teacher to make sure that the child accurately recorded the completed work, the daily work that he did not finish in school, and the assigned homework. The trick with this technique is making the child responsible for telling on himself. I find that if the child reports accurately, he will be in a better position to proceed with the unfinished work and the homework, and he is more likely to complete both kinds of assignments after school. If the child fails to write the information down, he is docked part of his allowance or other privileges. In some instances, it may be better to start with a smaller allowance and to reinforce the child by giving him an agreed-on bonus when he writes down the assignments correctly. After the child has mastered these tasks completely, the parents can often gradually withdraw the reinforcement and return to the usual allowance. After the notebook procedure has continued several weeks, the parents need only spot check with the teacher. However, as is the case for most responsibilities expected of most ADD children, the child should continue to use self-monitoring techniques long after his behavior is satisfactory. It is my impression that by really overdoing these techniques, parents can finally depend on the child to maintain some behavior patterns without such external supports.

Although this example involved school assignments, analogous procedures—with notebooks or calendars—can be worked out for such areas of the child's life as personal hygiene, grooming, music and dancing lessons, and so forth.

Special Psychological Help for the Family and Child

From time to time I have referred to the fact that in some families—either because of the presence of the ADD child or for entirely different reasons—there will be much family stress and strain. Such family difficulties cause problems for any child and they may cause greater problems for the ADD child. If the parents cannot agree between themselves as to rules for their children, if they do not consistently reward and punish, if they criticize one child or favor another because of their own personal problems, they will create psychological difficulties for their children. Obviously, families with disturbances need professional help, regardless of whether they have an ADD child, and this is the kind of situation in which help can be provided by psychiatrists, social workers, or psychologists. Any steps that will decrease difficulties within the family will be of special benefit to the ADD child, since adjustment to even ordinary social demands is already difficult for him. Even if he responds well to medication, he may not respond to emotional stress as flexibly as a child who does not have the problems associated with ADD.

Another form of specific psychological help that is *sometimes* useful for the ADD child is psychotherapy, in which the child meets with a therapist, either individually or with other children in a group. The purposes of psychotherapy are to enable a child to recognize and understand his feelings and to learn to deal with them appropriately. Psychotherapy, a very popular mode of treatment, has in the past been considered to be the best treatment for virtually all psychiatric difficulties both in adults and in children. Currently, however, one of the major questions in adult and child psychiatry concerns the effectiveness of psychotherapy for particular problems. There are no data whatsoever supporting the usefulness of psychotherapy in the basic treatment of ADD children. Nonetheless, many experienced psychiatrists have found that it is sometimes a useful auxiliary technique with some ADD children. In my own experience it has been most useful with older ADD children and especially with those older children who have "engrafted" psychological disabilities on their temperamental ones. Many of the difficulties of these children concern interpersonal relations, and it is my impression that psychotherapy has proved useful with some of these children some of the time. These have generally been ADD children who did not receive treatment with medication in their earlier years and as a result fell into the vicious circle of school and familial problems. They seem to have benefited from a relationship with a warm and impartial adult who was able to provide them with some understanding of their problems and help them in the construction of solutions to these problems.

Certainly individual psychotherapy is not the treatment of choice for most ADD children. Unfortunately, the usefulness of medication and the other techniques discussed has only recently been recognized. In the past many ADD children received psychotherapy, and for most of them it apparently was not helpful. Since it is a time-consuming and expensive procedure, it should only be used when there is a strong possibility that working with the child's special problems may be useful, or when the child seems unresponsive to all other forms of treatment. This is certainly an area of hot dispute and many psychiatrists would undoubtedly disagree with me. All I can state is that I have seen dozens of ADD children who have received psychotherapy, often for years, with no visible benefit, and who subsequently responded dramatically to treatment with medication. As repeatedly stated, the basis of most ADD children's problems is physiological and must be dealt with physiologically—that is, with the aid of medication. Medication goes to the root of the problem. Psychotherapy may help to deal with some of the branches that, so to speak, have grown in the wrong direction. Many parents do not feel this way. I remember one very sophisticated mother whose seriously afflicted ADD child had responded dramatically to medication. At the first visit after medication had been started the mother reported, "Tim is 100 percent better, Doctor. Now let's put him in psychotherapy and really get to the root of the problem."

Although psychotherapy is occasionally useful in some ADD children, simpler measures should be employed first. If medication, educational remediation, and parental counseling fail to help the child as much as seems necessary, psychotherapy can be tried.

Vacations for the Parents

Living with difficult children is difficult. The techniques I have discussed may make parents' lives easier, but their lives may still be much harder than those of most parents. For this reason I think that it is very important for the parents of ADD children to get away sometimes by themselves. (It is probably highly desirable for *all* parents. It is essential for the parents of ADD children.) It is not a sign of intellectual, moral, or physical weakness for these parents to want a periodic vacation alone. ADD children demand much attention, and caring for them can be physically, mentally, and emotionally exhausting. In addition, sometimes the parents' relationship suffers as a result of the tension surrounding the child's problems. The happiness and well-being of everyone should not be sacrificed for the good of the child with problems. Everyone deserves a piece of the pie. Thus, it is an excellent practice for parents to schedule regular time-out periods for themselves.

Obviously, such vacations pose practical problems. The ADD child is often too much of a handful to deposit with unsuspecting relatives. If the community has an organization for parents of ADD children, it might offer opportunities to share child care, with the parents taking turns at vacations without the children. Such trading has the advantage that all the adults involved are aware of the problems of the ADD child and have some knowledge of how to handle them. This kind of trading off is not just of selfish value to the parents. If they are able to spend some time alone with each other and enjoy themselves, they may be more relaxed in handling their ADD child when they return, which would benefit the child (and other children in the family as well). But whether or not this is the case, it is sufficient that the parents themselves will feel better.

EDUCATIONAL MANAGEMENT

ADD children frequently experience academic difficulties that seem to arise from two major sources. First, most ADD children are likely to have some problems in learning because of their distractibility, lack of stick-to-itiveness, readiness to give up, tendency to rush through things, and inability to discipline themselves (especially with respect to doing homework). *Some* ADD children also have the specific perceptual difficulties (reversals, etc.) that have been called learning disabilities and are now known as specific developmental disorders (SDD; see description in Chapter 2).

There are therefore two groups of ADD chidren with learning problems: (1) those whose learning problems are secondary only to distractibility and inattentiveness; and (2) those whose learning difficulties are secondary to these inattention difficulties and also to specific perceptual problems (SDD). Because of its effect on the child's overall organization and attentiveness, medication sometimes eliminates and frequently diminishes learning problems, particularly in the first group of children. However, even among those in whom the learning problems diminish with medication, additional educational assistance is often needed. Too often, by the time the ADD child's academic problems are recognized and treated, he has failed to master basic material and has fallen behind in many subjects. Learning problems are cumulative, even in children of normal or above normal intelligence. Consequently, the child cannot compensate for his educational losses, despite improved functioning, unless remedial or "catch-up" tutoring is provided in those areas in which he has fallen behind. The problem of cumulative educational lacks is most severe in those ADD children whose difficulties are first recognized in adolescence. They have often received social promotions and may be several grade levels behind in a number of subjects. Unfortunately, although medication may still be effective, appropriate educational facilities are often not available, and these children, frustrated and embarrassed by their poor academic showing, tend to give up.

The children with specific developmental disorder (SDD) are another problem. Medicine *may* improve their attention span and stick-to-itiveness but does not remedy their perceptual difficulties. Scientific experiments have shown that stimulant medication is no more effective than an inactive placebo in facilitating learning in children with reading problems. What is effective—to varying degrees—is special remedial education. However, although many people have investigated the teaching of "dyslexics," and many different approaches have been recommended by people with doctoral degrees in special education, there is no consensus about which children do best with which special education. Effective teaching can improve the reading and spelling performance of children with developmental disorders in reading, but with limits to the improvement that can be expected. Reading and spelling may continue to be problems as the child grows older, although the extent of the problem will vary, depending on the child's responsiveness, the nature of the teaching, the emphasis in the school, and the child's interests. For example, some private schools and a few public schools have been able to help children of normal intelligence with reading problems by the use of audiotaped materials and oral tests.

Similarly, developmental disorders in mathematics, which are compatible with excellent abstracting skill in higher mathematics, are now less of an academic handicap than they once were. The $5 calculator has been an enormous help to those who have difficulty in doing complex addition, multiplication, and division. If the child can master columnar arrangement and the placement of the decimal point, he can solve the problems. Being calculator-dependent may not be an asset, but it is certainly not a great liability.

Since many educators do not recognize ADD children as a unique category, they frequently place such children in special educational classes, even though they have no specific perceptual problems. In addition, many children placed in these classes have both ADD problems and perceptual difficulties. In both types a trial of medication is generally useful. To repeat, there is no way of predicting a child's response, and one may anticipate that some problems will disappear whereas others (including the perceptual ones) may remain. Any child who has been placed in a special class without a specific diagnosis of his difficulties should be carefully evaluated to see if he has ADD problems and is therefore eligible for a trial of medication.

It may be useful to mention some educational approaches that have been tried but have not demonstrated effectiveness. A number of people had noticed that some children had both learning and coordination problems. (Approximately half of ADD children do have some coordination difficulties.) These people reasoned, erroneously, that the learning problems were probably the result of the coordination problems. (Both are probably the result of a third factor.) They also believed that training in coordination might improve the learning difficulties. For this reason they prescribed exercises, involving either the whole body or the eyes. *At present there is no evidence whatsoever that coordination training will help the ADD child's learning difficulties.* The same statement applies to specific treatment programs of eye exercises.

However, coordination training *may* help the ADD child's coordination problems. The coordination difficulties from which many ADD children suffer are frequently embarrassing or humiliating to the child. This is particularly true for boys. To be chosen last when teams are being picked and to be ridiculed for athletic inadequacy are blows to the ADD boy's already shaky self-esteem. There are programs in physical reeducation—not readily available—in which the children receive specific tutoring in motor tasks of increasing difficulty. My impression is that these programs sometimes improve the child's coordination and generally increase his self-confidence. If such programs are not available, the parent may help the poorly coordinated ADD child by guiding him toward physical activity in which fine coordination presents less of a problem. As mentioned, many ADD children have particular problems with hand-eye coordination and as a result are worst in such sports as baseball and tennis. Sometimes they encounter less difficulty in football—particularly in line play, where gross body movement is required—or in basketball. These children may often perform adequately or excellently in sports requiring large muscle control, such as running or swimming. Judo also seems a good sport for the ADD child; even though he may not do as well as the non-ADD child, he can acquire skills that give him the novel feeling of being a "big man," a feeling that often considerably bolsters his self-esteem.

SPECIAL PROBLEMS OF ADOLESCENCE

The ADD child whose problem is first discovered in adolescence poses several practical problems. The first is that he already has had years of unhappy experience as a result of his attention deficit disorder. The second major problem is that adolescence is a time of rebellion for most children, ADD or otherwise. Since the child is now increasingly independent, his cooperation in the treatment program is absolutely necessary. Furthermore, the behavioral techniques discussed are more useful with preadolescent children.

Most clinicians who treat many ADD patients find that it is much easier to treat an adolescent who has been treated and followed since childhood than it is to work with an adolescent who has never been treated before. This is quite understandable if one thinks of some of the major psychological issues of adolescence. If an adolescent is diagnosed as having ADD and if medication is recommended, think of what problems may follow. In general, the adolescent is not complaining himself. Like the ADD child, he is brought to the doctor because he is not doing well and (probably) causing problems for others. But the adolescent feels that he is different—that he has different tastes, values, wishes—and that treatment is being recommended not because he has a disorder but because he is not the way his parents would like him to be. Another issue is self-esteem. The adolescent's self-esteem is always shaky, and the ADD adolescent's self-esteem is even worse. Learning that he may have to take medicine for a condition of which he was unaware (ADD) can be another blow.

The difficulties in treating the adolescent for the first time are not insurmountable, but they do cause serious problems. If the adolescent can be convinced that the medication is something that is being done for him rather than to him, his cooperation can sometimes be obtained. Similarly, if he can be convinced that medication will give him more freedom by giving him more control of himself, he may be more willing to take it. Otherwise, he is likely to see medication as a chemical straitjacket employed by an oppressive adult world to control someone whose views differ. If he can be persuaded that medication will help him to control himself, he may accept its use. Unfortunately, without previous experience with the medication, he cannot know that it will enable him to control his temper if he wants to control it, and that he can still remain rebellious if he chooses to do so. He finds it difficult to understand that improved concentration will enable him to do better at studying subjects he is interested in—although of course he may still object to having to study some of the required parts of the curriculum.

Because of these problems in treating an ADD adolescent for the first time, clinicians much prefer to treat ADD symptoms when they become a problem in childhood. Treatment in childhood does not prevent symptoms in adolescence, but early experience with medication and with the therapist enables the child to understand that medication may help him and that the therapist can be a friend who is not an agent of his parents. If that child still requires medication in adolescence, he accepts it much more readily.

On the positive side of the ledger, the adolescent is in a better position to understand and recognize the basis of his difficulties. This understanding, if it can be obtained, may balance out the other problems. From a practical standpoint, helping the adolescent ADD child generally requires the treating physician to spend more time in seeing the adolescent individually, or often with his family as part of family therapy.

If the ADD adolescent has had serious learning problems, the situation may be critical. If he is five years behind in reading and spelling, school will be a nightmare. It is often difficult and sometimes impossible to convince such an adolescent that he is not a "retard." If he can be convinced that he has reading problems that are not associated with intelligence and that he is not a moron, half the battle has been won. The second half is more difficult to accomplish. He must be entered in some kind of program in which his abilities will allow him to succeed and in which his disabilities will not seriously penalize him. If the public schools available to the youngster do not have the flexibility to help him explore the areas in which he might do well, it might be desirable for the parents to look for a private school that offers more options.

SUMMARY

In capsule form I would like to repeat the major points of this chapter.

First, most ADD children respond to medication. *All* ADD children deserve a trial of medication since there is absolutely no way of predicting which children will respond well and which children will not. Sometimes medication alone is enough. Since the prescription of medication requires a doctor, a physician must always be involved in the treatment of the ADD child.

Second, changes in the relationship between the parents and the ADD child are almost always helpful. Understanding and the establishment of firm, consistent, explicit, predictable rules are always useful. Frequently, these can be achieved with little or no professional help yet sometimes the assistance of a psychiatrist, psychologist, or social worker may be helpful.

Third, some ADD children need special educational assistance. In many instances this will only involve remedial education, while in some instances it may mean special education.

With such interventions, most ADD children can be helped, often to a substantial degree. Not only will these forms of intervention diminish the present problems of ADD children, but also they will often help to prevent future ones.

6

Attention Deficit Disorder in Adults

ATTENTION DEFICIT DISORDER—DOES IT EXIST IN ADULTS?

Until recently, most child psychiatrists believed that ADD diminished in adolescence and disappeared in adulthood. Although this pattern does hold for more than half of the ADD children, there is increasing reason to believe that some children continue to have a variety of ADD symptoms as adults.

Prior to recent evidence, a few physicians who had treated hyperactive (ADD) patients in childhood and adolescence, and then in later life, noticed the persistence of some symptoms as the children became adults. Throughout this time these patients also showed the same response to stimulant medication, finding it calming and beneficial.

Physicians used to believe that the reaction of ADD children to stimulant medication was paradoxical. Whereas stimulants usually produce euphoria and excitement in adults, they seem to produce quietness and settling down in ADD children. It is not clear whether this is true of other children because no one has given stimulant drugs to non-ADD children over a period of weeks or months. However, when non-ADD children with learning disabilities are given stimulant drugs, they do not calm down but often become anxious, irritable, and driven. The common clinical belief was that as ADD children outgrew their problems in adolescence, the paradoxical response went away and that then the formerly ADD adolescents and adults responded to stimulant medications in the normal way.

The reports of clinicians who noticed that adults, too, could benefit from stimulant medication were generally neglected. Why? Beliefs arise in psychiatry either because many nonscientific clinicians observe the same phenomena over and over again or because scientific studies affirm and demonstrate the clinicians' observations. Twenty years ago clinicians who treated hyperactivity (ADD) in childhood were just beginning to observe its course systematically and frequently they disagreed. Psychiatry was nowhere near as scientific then as it is now, and child psychiatry was even less scientific—that is, no child psychiatrists were conducting careful studies in which they traced the development and outcome of a large group of ADD children.

During the past ten years, considerable evidence has accumulated indicating that ADD frequently persists into adolescence and into young adult life. Earlier, discussing the outcome of ADD with age, I mentioned some of this evidence. The studies began with carefully diagnosed ADD children and followed large numbers of them (100 in one study) from elementary school age to the late teen-age years; other studies looked at the outcome of a less-well-diagnosed group of ADD children who were followed well into their twenties. The evidence has been strong enough so that now there is an "official" way to diagnose ADD in adults.

In diagnosing patients, psychiatrists employ a manual that specifies the exact characteristics of psychiatric disorders. This manual now recognizes not only ADD and specific developmental disorders (SDD) but also ADD persisting into adult life. The official designation for the adult form of ADD is attention deficit disorder, residual type (ADD,RT)—that is, attention deficit disorder leaving a residue. The manual states that if the symptom of hyperactivity is present in childhood ADD it tends to disappear, but the other major symptoms of

ADD—concentration problems, impulsivity, and so forth—may persist. How common this is and what the other symptoms are in adults are not clearly stated because evidence was just beginning to accumulate on ADD,RT when the manual was published in 1980.

Information on the persistence of attention deficit disorder into adult life has also come from psychiatric case reports of individual patients with different diagnoses who had had ADD as children. The ADD problems seemed to be present to some extent in the adults; in some instances they changed with age. Very few of these case studies included investigations of the effects of stimulant medication.

For the past ten years, studies that I have conducted with my collaborators, Drs. Frederick Reimherr and David Wood, have expanded the information available on ADD,RT. We have carefully observed the effects of various treatments on approximately 150 patients whom we believe to be hyperactive children grown up—that is, adults with continuing problems of ADD. Reports on our work have been judged by editorial boards consisting of experts in this field, have been published in scientific journals, and have convinced many other clinicians that ADD may indeed persist into the thirties, forties, and fifties, and that in many instances it responds to stimulant medication in a way similar to the response in ADD children.

Several extremely important questions remain. The first is how common ADD is in adults. The second is what its distinguishing symptoms are. In our research, we have listed the symptoms we believe are present in adults with ADD. Before I describe them, I want to emphasize that research such as we have performed must be confirmed by other psychiatric researchers before it can be widely accepted. We have employed all the techniques customarily used to reduce chances of self-deceit—that is, to reduce the chances of our persuading ourselves that what we expect to find is true. However, the help of other psychiatric researchers is needed not only to confirm our findings but also to aid in independently identifying the symptoms of ADD in adults. Their help is particularly necessary for sorting out ADD,RT symptoms that are very similar to and can be confused with those of biological (chemical) depressions.

I am including this section on ADD in adults, even though it presents material that is not yet confirmed scientific knowledge, both because it may shed light on the child's later development and because it may be applicable to the parents reading this book. Since ADD clearly runs in families, the parents of the children and adolescents discussed are more likely to have had ADD in childhood than people in general. If such parents recognize in themselves the signs and symptoms indicated below, they may want to try the treatments we have investigated. However, although the first part of this book presents views widely accepted by child psychiatrists about ADD in children and adolescents, I must repeat that information in this section is tentative.

THE SYMPTOMS OF ADD IN ADULTS (ADD, RESIDUAL TYPE)

Overt Symptoms

The symptoms I am going to discuss are those that my colleagues and I used as we explored this disorder. Because the study of ADD,RT is comparatively recent, ideas about the symptoms themselves are still changing.

The first requirement for having a diagnosis of ADD in adulthood is that the person *must* have had it in childhood. That is, beginning before the age of seven, the child had the following persistent symptoms of inattentive and impulsive behavior (as described in Chapter 2). The following items are taken from the *Diagnostic and Statistical Manual of the American Psychiatric Association*, 3rd edition (known as DSM-III) and are the current defining characteristics necessary for a diagnosis of ADDH in childhood.

• *Inattention*: (1) often failed to finish things he or she started; (2) often didn't seem to listen; (3) easily distracted; (4) had difficulty concentrating on schoolwork or other tasks requiring sustained attention; (5) had difficulty sticking to a play activity.

• *Impulsivity*: (1) often acted before thinking; (2) shifted excessively from one activity to another; (3) had difficulty organizing work (not because of cognitive impairment); (4) needed a lot of supervision; (5) frequently called out in class; (6) had difficulty awaiting turn in games or group situations.

In addition, most—but not all—ADD,RT adults had the following symptoms of hyperactivity when they were children: (1) ran about or climbed on things excessively; (2) had difficulty sitting still or fidgeted excessively; (3) had difficulty staying seated; (4) moved about excessively during sleep; (5) was always on the go or acted as if driven by a motor.

However—and this is a big however—children with other psychiatric problems may have the same problems of inattentiveness, impulsivity, and hyperactivity. Therefore, even if an adult behaved this way as a child, a diagnosis of ADD,RT can be made *only* if those childhood symptoms clearly were not produced by any other form of psychiatric disorder.

Attention problems

Our patients experience the same sorts of problems with *attentiveness* that we have observed in children. They are often able to concentrate on material they're interested in but are not able to concentrate on what doesn't interest them. This is true even if the uninteresting things are important. They could not concentrate on fractions as a child. They cannot concentrate on the income tax form as adults. When this problem is severe, they may find it very difficult to read. The inattentiveness often causes difficulties at college, at work, and in other situations where attention is required for learning. The symptom is often present socially as well, and frequently they are unable to keep their mind on conversations. All psychiatrists working with couples have many times heard the complaint that the spouse does not listen; at times this may result from ADD,RT. Thus, another consequence of the inattentiveness can be disturbed social relationships.

Patients often complain of *distractibility*. One man who was a historian and also a novelist reported that the following kinds of experiences kept him from working when he sat down in his study: first he would hear the refrigerator go on; next he would respond to the cat coming through the door; then he would be disturbed by the continuing rustling of leaves on the roof. Being constantly distracted by such stimuli made writing extremely difficult. When he was later treated with stimulant medication, he reported that not only could he focus on his work but he was able to shut out such distracting noises.

Hyperactivity

Although hyperactivity is not necessary for the diagnosis of ADD in childhood, and often disappears as the child grows older, we have studied only those individuals who had been hyperactive as children and continue to show hyperactivity as adults. In this early phase of the investigation of ADD,RT we have used this restrictive definition because we wanted to study the most definite—and perhaps extreme—cases. We have done this because we wanted to reduce the risk of studying and treating people whose symptoms look like those of ADD but in fact are produced by other disorders.

When hyperactivity persists into adult life, it takes a somewhat different form from that in childhood. Of course our adults do not go running around classrooms anymore, but they are still frequently out of their seats. Often they report a nervousness. What they mean is not that they are anxious or worrying but that they grow impatient when sedentary activities are prolonged. They find it difficult to remain seated while watching a movie or TV, reading a newspaper, or studying at college. They feel a strong urge to get up and walk around. They feel more comfortable while being on the go, and they feel uncomfortable when forced to be inactive. Many of them have become fidgeters. We have had the repeated experience of identifying a new patient in the waiting room because he or she is continuously tapping on the arm of a chair or, more noticeably, jiggling a foot. During our diagnostic interviews we often find such patients squirming in the chair, tapping their legs, playing with their hands, or picking at their face and hair.

All the patients we have defined as having residual ADD have been hyperactive and inattentive. In addition, for a diagnosis of ADD,RT we require that they have two or more of the following symptoms. Again, it is important to emphasize that neither we nor other investigators are sure that these symptoms correctly identify ADD,RT or that any particular number of them should be present for a definite diagnosis.

Impulsivity

Our patients describe difficulties in self-control. They have a tendency to act first and think second. They have difficulty tolerating frustration and often act to relieve that frustration instead of thinking things through carefully. They tend to do things on the spur of the moment and regret their actions later. They do not like postponing decisions and, because they do not think things out, they often do not anticipate fairly obvious consequences of their actions. Socially, like ADD children, they tend to interrupt when other people are talking.

The negative consequences of impulsivity are greater for adults than for children. Whereas running on the playground may result in only a teacher's reprimand, reckless speeding or gambling often have more serious consequences. Looking only at present pleasure and avoiding thoughts of future pain, adults with ADD,RT can be impulse buyers, initiators of foolish business activities, and participants in short-lived romances and marriages.

Mood swings

Another area in which difficulties are often seen is mood. Our ADD,RT patients describe problems with mood that frequently go back as far as they can remember, often before adolescence. What they tell us is that their mood changes frequently. They describe being very reactive—that is, they tend to become depressed much more readily and to a greater degree than other people when they encounter frustration, loss, or defeat. They also tend to shift in the opposite direction. They will describe becoming excited and overstimulated when things go well, and they distinguish this feeling from genuine happiness. It seems to be the adult equivalent of the overexcitement one sees in ADD children in stimulating environments, such as the supermarket or the circus. As they get older, the excited periods seem to occur less often. Their moods come and go quickly. Their downs can be relieved by a change in circumstances. Our patients have also told us that their moods frequently shift by themselves for no apparent reason. Their ups and downs last a few hours or at most a few days. When they do last for longer periods, it is because the patients have "dug themselves into holes" in life. The depression is described as being "down," "bored," or "discontented"—and frequently the patients distinguish it from sadness.

Disorganization and inability to complete tasks

Our patients describe difficulty in organizing their lives in both minor and major ways. They are disorganized in solving problems, and they are disorganized in structuring their time. They tell us that at home and at work they frequently move from one task to another before completing the first one. Because of such planlessness and shifting around, they often report that it takes them much longer than it should to complete projects. The kind of shifting they describe is not what we all adopt to avoid boredom (I'll read this book for an hour, then balance the checkbook, and then prepare dinner). They recall having jumbled desks at school, and if they are white-collar workers they now have trouble setting priorities and finding what they need in their desks and files. At home, they may find it difficult to pay bills on time or to keep track of tools. If they continue with school, their efforts are hamstrung by the same disorganization they had as children.

It is important, however, to distinguish this tendency to jump from one thing to another, which may be a facet of impulsivity, from a realistic response to the multiple pressures of a busy daily life. For example, a well-organized woman who has young children, is employed, and takes care of her own home often cannot complete all she would like to do in any one day, but this has no relation to ADD,RT.

In contrast, the lack of ability to plan activities adequately is the characteristic that may be a symptom of ADD in an adult.

Short and hot temper

During childhood, many but not all ADD children are described as having a low boiling point or a short fuse. As children they may have had more than their share of temper tantrums and fights at school. The ADD adults we have seen tend to have short-lived anger. They explode but do not brood or nurse anger. With age, some have learned how to count to ten, while others have learned that for them the only effective technique for avoiding an explosion is to leave the scene. Temper outbursts sometimes produce the most serious problems patients have to face. Bad temper may cost them jobs, destroy personal relationships (including marriage), distance them from their children, and end friendships.

Low stress tolerance

Finally, we also see in the adults with ADD an overreactivity that is a hard attribute to measure but very important to our patients. They describe themselves as having a chronically thin skin. They become easily flustered, hassled, tense, or uptight. They perceive themselves as making mountains out of molehills and becoming readily distressed, and they frequently find themselves psychologically incapacitated. Overreacting to stress also increases their difficulties in solving their problems, which makes a bad situation worse. It also produces a vicious circle because failure to solve problems increases tension, which results in a decreased ability to solve problems, and so forth.

Heredity and ADD,RT Symptoms

In addition to such symptoms, certain patterns of behavior within the family may suggest the diagnosis of ADD,RT in an adult. If John and Mary Doe have an ADD child and Mary clearly does not have ADD or a history of ADD in the family, the odds increase that John is carrying the disorder and may also have some symptoms himself. Similarly, if an adult is having the above problems and has a parent or brothers or sisters with similar problems, he should consider the possibility that he may have ADD,RT. In years past, neither one's siblings nor one's parents would be formally diagnosed as having ADD,RT. But since the symptoms of ADD are so obvious, it is possible to make an educated guess about the diagnosis. If a relative is continually restless, distracted, disorganized, hot-tempered, impulsive, and moody, the chances that he has ADD,RT are fairly high.

Psychological Problems with ADD,RT

Our ADD,RT patients frequently have special psychological problems. Not surprisingly, these are often continuations of similar problems in childhood. The hyperactive adults we have studied tend to be obstinate, bossy, strong willed, and stubborn. This does not make them easy to live with. Because of the problems I have already mentioned, the adults, like the children, tend to be underachievers at work and in the home and they continue to have interpersonal difficulties. As a result of numerous unsatisfying experiences, they often have low self-esteem. As one patient who was a baseball fan observed, when your life is characterized by no hits, no runs, and plenty of errors, you do not have a terrific view of yourself.

The patients tend to be dissatisfied with their lives in general. Their impulsivity, their temper, and perhaps the same sort of social obtuseness seen in the children disturb their personal lives. Relationships tend to be stormy, and we suspect that break-ups of relationships and marriages are more common than in patients without ADD. On the job they not only fail to obtain promotions but tend to be fired frequently because of their disorganization and hot temper.

Specific developmental disorders (SDDs) also often persist, and ADD,RT adults have more than their share of difficulties in reading, spelling, and arithmetic. Confusion of right and left may also continue, along with reversal in numbers and letters. Obviously, problems of this kind can easily interfere with performance in a variety of different jobs.

At the expense of being repetitious, I wish to emphasize that psychiatrists do not agree on how many and which of these symptoms must be present to reach a diagnosis of ADD in adults. Further, many of the symptoms I have just enumerated are seen in a variety of other psychiatric disorders. Even if a person is hyperactive and inattentive and has several of the other problems listed, he or she may have another psychiatric disorder. Symptoms very similar to these are seen in adults who have depressions that are considered biological in origin (such depressions are believed to result from faulty body chemistry, to be frequently hereditary, and to respond to treatment with medication far better than they do to psychological treatment). Obviously, anyone who has at least four of the problems I listed does indeed have problems that suggest the advisability of psychiatric evaluation. He or she may not have adult ADD but would probably benefit by appropriate treatment of some kind.

DIAGNOSIS OF ADULT ADD

One of the difficulties in diagnosing adults is that they often do not remember what they were like as children. In our research, we have dealt with this problem in two ways: we have instructed prospective patients to talk with their parents about the patients' problems during childhood, and we have requested the parents of prospective patients to fill out questionnaires describing the psychological characteristics and problems that the patients had when they were children. For both the diagnosis and the evaluation of treatment, it is extremely important to have the help of the spouse, significant other, or parent of the adult with possible ADD.

The parents of ADD children painfully recognize that the children either do not perceive or will acknowledge the basis of their problems. The children may agree that they are not doing well in school or that they are having difficulty with peers, siblings, or their parents, but they rarely acknowledge responsibility for these problems (or the role that their behavior plays in causing these problems). The same imperceptiveness is often seen in ADD adults. Partly it may be due to psychological self-protection. Not only do we not like to disclose our problems to other people, but we do not like to disclose them to ourselves. Failure to perceive one's problems is a psychological protection method used not only by individuals with psychiatric difficulties of various kinds but also by most of the rest of the world as well. Another reason that the ADD adult may be blind to his psychological imperfections is that he has lived his whole life with them. In contrast, individuals who develop psychiatric disorders recognize the changes immediately: They will tell us how and when they felt depressed, became anxious, or lost control of their temper. But the ADD adult has always lived with his problems. He is like someone who is color-blind— he does not realize he is different because he has always been that way.

Because of the difficulty of recognizing ADD,RT and of distinguishing it from other disorders, it is important that someone with problems of this kind not attempt to diagnose himself. The above descriptions are designed to serve as a list of warning symptoms that can alert the reader to the presence of problems that should be evaluated by a trained professional.

DRUG TREATMENT OF THE ADD ADULT

As with the ADD child, medication is the most effective treatment for adults with ADD,RT. When medication works, and it does so in about two-thirds of our patients, the effects are often dramatic. Many patients in our experimental programs had received treatment with both medication and psychotherapy before we had seen them. Because the symptoms of adult ADD are similar in some respects to certain types of depressions, the patients had been given the standard medications employed in depression (the tricyclic antidepressants, which I mentioned, and lithium). In general, they had not been treated with the two types of medications we have found most effective: stimulant drugs and the monoamine oxidase inhibitors. Other drugs are also sometimes used, but these two types are the chief therapeutic agents.

Stimulant Drugs

The stimulant drugs we have found most useful are the amphetamines, methylphenidate, and pemoline. When effective, these drugs produce the following effects.

Effects

Inattentiveness and distractibility. Both these characteristics are reduced by the stimulant medications. Responding patients find they can focus their attention better on academic and office work, reading for pleasure, television, and movies. In addition, they are able to attend more to what others are saying, and are more sensitive to mood and attitude changes in others. Since bad listening skills are a frequent cause of marital and family discord, being able to pay better attention to what others say and to what others want and don't want cannot help improving interpersonal relations. Increased attentiveness of this kind is not a paradoxical response. Anyone who takes stimulant medications in low doses may report that he concentrates better, and this may affect how he approaches necessary tasks. However, in contrast to the effect on the ADD,RT adult, it is not clear how useful this is for the normal person. For example, typists do not type faster and more accurately on amphetamines.

Hyperactivity. When present, fidgetiness, restlessness, and discomfort at being sedentary all disappear. Fingers stop tapping, feet stop jiggling, and the treated patient will report that he can sit through a TV program or a movie with much greater ease. At the same time, overall physical and mental energy is not decreased.

Impulsivity. The decrease in impulsivity can be observed in a small way on a day-to-day basis and also over a longer period of time. Patients successfully treated with stimulants think before they talk—they "engage their mind before they put their mouth in gear." They also converse more usefully. The ADD child and adult frequently interrupt—they cannot wait to get their words in. When medication is effective, arguments about not being listened to or not being heard out decrease. Impulsivity toward children changes: parents scream and hit less. Because sudden surges of feeling are less likely, the chances of strained or broken relationships also diminish. Impulse buying, spending sprees, and perhaps certain compulsive-impulsive activities such as gambling decrease. To a greater extent, the patient considers the consequences of his behavior and acts accordingly.

Mood problems. When effective, medication removes both the highs and the lows. The normal person who takes amphetamines is likely to become euphoric—that is, he may develop an inappropriate intense feeling of pleasure (as in some mental illnesses). Such euphoria can lead to possible misuse and addiction. The ADD,RT patient, however, does not become euphoric: he is less bored, less discontented, and happier with his lot, but he is not euphoric.

Organization. Patients improve their planning. Students, homemakers, and wage earners begin to devote more thought to the organization of their daily activities. One sees such concrete results as homework and papers completed on time, improved regulation of children's activities, better meal preparation, better care of house and yard, prompt bill payment, and improved meeting of job deadlines. As a result, relations improve with both spouses and employers.

Hot temper. Effective treatment lengthens the fuse and raises the boiling point—successfully treated patients explode less frequently and more mildly. The effects on a household may be profound. Since ADD children tend to have ADD parents, the common family situation is a tense one—a very difficult child and a short-tempered parent. The best management of ADD children requires planning and coolness, and the ADD parent is poorly equipped to deal with an ADD child. Temper control and the organizational changes already mentioned can help greatly. Even though the hot temper of ADD adults tends to be short lived, no one enjoys having to live with a person who cannot control himself. Again, interpersonal relations improve.

Management of stress.   Successfully treated ADD adults report that their stress tolerance goes up—that they are less easily hassled or discombobulated. The continuing stresses and strains of everyday life make them less anxious, less depressed, and less confused. This obviously plays a role in their demonstrable better organization. It is hard to follow a plan systematically when your motivation and mood change from moment to moment.

Dosage

The dosages that have proved effective in ADD adults are approximately the same as those that have been useful for children. In most instances the doses of *d*-amphetamine (Dexedrine) have been between 10 and 40 mg/day, of methylphenidate between 20 and 80 mg/day, and pemoline between 37.5 and 150 mg/day. As previously mentioned, in the nonlong-acting forms, pemoline is effective for the longest period of time, the amphetamines for an intermediate period, and methylphenidate for the least time. If the useful effect of a medication is only 1½ to 2 hours, the patient may have to take eight doses a day to achieve a good therapeutic effect. Since this is obviously unsatisfactory, the treating physician will attempt to substitute a longer-acting drug or a dosage form intended to last for 8 to 12 hours (but does not always do so).

Side effects

The most common side effects are appetite loss and, if the medication is taken too late in the day, difficulty in falling asleep. The appetite loss and the resulting weight loss are short lived, and after several weeks the patient's appetite returns to normal. The sleep-inhibiting effects, however, do not disappear with time. A common problem is that the therapeutic effect of the medication wears off while the arousing effect remains. For example, a dose of *d*-amphetamine taken at 4:00 PM might provide psychological benefits till 9:00 or 10:00 PM but keep the individual up long past midnight. One alternative is to take the last dose earlier in the day, but that means that good effects disappear in the late afternoon and early evening. Another alternative is to give a small dose of a sedative major tranquilizer (thioridazine, as described in the section on drug treatment for children) an hour before bedtime. This appears to counteract the arousing effect of the stimulant drug without interfering with its beneficial action the next day.

Special problems

Two major problems exist with stimulant medication, one medical and the other legal. The medical problem is that the medication does not work before the patient takes it in the morning and wears off before he goes to sleep at night. If he is a very difficult person to live with (e.g., with an explosive temper), then even with drug treatment there are still likely to be several bad hours a day, early in the morning and late in the evening. The patients themselves obviously do not like this roller coaster effect. It can sometimes be avoided by the use of monoamine oxidase inhibitors, which I describe below.

The second major problem with the amphetamines and methylphenidate—and pemoline to a much lesser degree—is that they can be abused. The amphetamines—"speed"—can produce powerful feelings of excitation and euphoria when taken in large doses, particularly when injected into a vein. Because serious drug abuse problems developed in the late 1960s, the federal government developed a policy regulating the prescription of drugs that can be abused or produce addiction. Drugs are placed in four categories, with the highest representing the most abusable medications. Amphetamines and methylphenidate have been placed in the same category as morphine, which means that they can be prescribed for only one month at a time (with no refills), written prescriptions must be used rather than telephone orders, and in many states copies of the prescription must be filed in duplicate or triplicate.

This understandable regulation complicates the medical management of ADD,RT. The amphetamines have been used in the practice of medicine since the 1930s. Whether wisely prescribed or not, many individuals took fixed doses for long periods of time, claimed to benefit from them, and did not increase the dose taken. Although amphetamines were occasionally abused, the epidemic of amphetamine abuse did not begin until the hippy era of the 1960s. To obtain the desired effects, the amphetamine or methylphenidate abuser must escalate the dosage. Eventually, some amphetamine addicts have taken several hundred milligrams several times a day over a period of several days. The doses they employ per day may be ten to one hundred times as great as those used therapeutically in the treatment of ADD. Methylphenidate has been abused much less than the amphetamines, either because it is less desirable or less readily available. Pemoline is insoluble in water and cannot be administered by vein. The important scientific question here is whether the ADD adult who might benefit from the comparatively low doses of amphetamine and methylphenidate that are useful therapeutically might obtain the highs associated with abuse if he took much larger doses or used the drugs intravenously. Unfortunately, we have no information with which to answer this question.

Because amphetamine and methylphenidate are known as highly abusable drugs, psychiatrists and other physicians are reluctant to use them in adults. That is one of the reasons our ADD adults were treated with other agents rather than stimulants before they were referred to us. Because ADD adults are impulsive, and many have had more than their share of troubles with abuse of alcohol and other drugs (such as marijuana), the physician is particularly reluctant to prescribe a drug that is commonly thought of in terms of possible abuse. Thus, ironically, ADD adults are least likely to be treated with the drugs that in our experience have been most effective—the stimulant drugs.

Monoamine Oxidase Inhibitors

Monoamine oxidase inhibitors (MAOIs) are a family of drugs developed over twenty years ago for the treatment of serious depressions (they and the tricyclic antidepressants are the two major categories of antidepressants). Like stimulants, they are less frequently used than they should be.

Effects

When effective, the action of the MAOIs is similar, though not identical, to that seen with the stimulants. There are several differences. First, their action is not immediate. The medication is typically begun at a low dose and increased over time, and it may be as long as two weeks after the best dose is reached before therapeutic effects appear. As the medication is continued, added benefit occurs, and it may take six to eight weeks before the drugs are fully effective. Unlike stimulants, the drugs act 24 hours a day. Their effect on patients varies: for some it tends to be stimulating and for others sedative. Accordingly, instructions to patients vary. Patients who are stimulated take them morning and noon, while patients who find them sedative may take them in the afternoon and evening.

Dosage

The MAOIs that our group has used are pargyline (Eutonyl), in dosages of 30 to 150 mg/day, and tranylcypromine (Parnate), in dosages of 10 to 60 mg/day. Because some slight tolerance to the MAOIs can occur over time, the dose may have to be increased slightly. As with the stimulants, it might be necessary to rotate MAOIs, shifting from one to another if tolerance develops.

Side effects

There is one major and potentially dangerous side effect from the MAOIs. Because of this side effect, they have been less frequently used than the tricyclic antidepressants. If certain foods or drugs are taken with MAOIs, a dangerous elevation of blood pressure may occur. The safe use of MAOIs requires that the patient abstain from certain foods and that he check out medications—including over-the-counter medications—before taking them. Prohibited foods include Stilton cheese and aged cheese, some alcoholic beverages (particularly port, chianti, other red wines, sherries, and beer), broad bean pods, canned figs, chicken livers, chocolate or coffee in large amounts, licorice, pickled herring, raisins, salted fish, sauerkraut, snails, soy sauce, and yeast products. These foods are banned to be on the safe side, but conclusive clinical evidence linking foods and elevation of blood pressure has indicted only aged cheeses and red wines. It is possible to have an interesting and varied diet while observing these limitations.

The other major side effect of the MAOIs is a reduction in blood pressure, particularly when standing up suddenly. This problem can be avoided in most instances by slowly increasing and adjusting the dose.

Thus, MAOIs offer medication that lasts 24 hours a day and is not abusable, but physicians are reluctant to use them because of the dangerous side effects if used incautiously. Which type of medication an individual patient responds to best can only be determined by trying both stimulants and MAOIs. Obviously, if someone does very well on the first medication tried, there is no reason to try another.

Judging Response to Medication

Like children with ADD, adults with ADD,RT do not recognize their problems initially and then may fail to notice their progress after treatment. As indicated in the following anecdotes, the judgment of another person is highly desirable in measuring improvement.

Some months following our completion of a controlled study of pemoline, I was stopped in the hall of the medical center by a nurse I did not know. She introduced herself and said, "I'd like to thank you very much." I replied: "You're welcome. What did I do?" It turned out that her husband had participated in the drug study, and that the medication had had a beneficial effect on their marriage. It had been deteriorating over several years and, despite counseling, the couple had been rapidly approaching divorce. The nurse stated that the stimulant medication had produced a pronounced change in her husband's behavior, and with its help they had been able to iron out their chronic problems. I had not treated the patient and asked his treating physician about him. Although we generally query others in our drug studies, that had been impossible in this instance because the nurse was away caring for her sick mother during the time of the drug trial. The treating physician had rated the patient as slightly improved—by the patient's judgment. By the wife's judgment, however, there had been marked improvement.

The same phenomenon occurred in my treatment of another patient. Each week, I reviewed the core symptoms of ADD and asked the patient whether or not he had improved, worsened, or stayed the same. One week, when both the patient and his wife had come to see me, he answered my questions about restlessness, inattentiveness, organization, and temper by saying that he was slightly improved. His overall judgment was also that he was "slightly improved." When he said this, his wife looked at him in surprise, placed her hand on his knee, and said to both of us, "Slightly better! It's like being married to a different man!"

In both of these cases, the patients' inaccurate self-observation was the adult equivalent of the ADD child's lack of awareness of his problems and of the change in behavior in response to medication.

When and How Long to Treat with Medication

The question of when to treat with medication arises because ADD problems can be present in differing amounts. Both serious and milder symptoms may respond to treatment. The practical questions are how much benefit is achieved with medication and what the risks are of its long-term use. Cost-benefit questions of this kind, of course, frequently occur in other areas of life as well as in medicine. To the best of our current knowledge, the risks incurred by long-term treatment with stimulant medication are very low. In the era before restrictions were placed on the use of stimulant medications, tens of millions of people took them without addiction, and no epidemic of serious problems was reported. So far as allergies and unusual reactions are concerned, the amphetamines and methylphenidate appear to be much safer than aspirin or penicillin. Allergic reactions are so uncommon that doctors who treat children with these medications have abandoned periodic blood testing to detect allergy. Still, the medications do increase heart rate, and in some individuals they raise blood pressure slightly. What happens to patients treated with these drugs for an extended period? It is impossible to answer this question in a straightforward way, since failure to treat may cause far greater stresses, such as loss of jobs, termination of relationships, frustrations, depression, and alcohol abuse. These and other consequences of untreated ADD may have far worse effects on the body than those resulting from the medications.

From a practical standpoint, clinicians who treat patients with ADD find that they tend to request treatment when their lives have become difficult, take medicine and with its help straighten out their lives, and then discontinue medication until the next emergency arises. This may not be the wisest policy for an ADD adult to follow because he is frequently unaware of the effects of his disorder on others; he may be destroying personal relationships, producing family turmoil, and impairing job success without awareness. Periodic use of medication is a good idea if the patient and his significant other learn to recognize when his supposedly mild ADD is causing problems that he does not usually perceive. The basic policy for the ADD patient should be to make sure his problems are not hurting himself and others. To determine this, he may need the help of others.

PSYCHOLOGICAL THERAPIES FOR THE ADD ADULT

The first essential component in the psychological treatment of the ADD adult is education. The patient must learn to recognize which symptoms of ADD cause him difficulties and must learn to observe them in his daily life. Just as a significant other is very important for diagnosis, so this other is extremely valuable in treatment. If he or she knows the patient well, a spouse or other partner will be able to recognize the subtleties of the patient's problems and response to treatment.

Although most of us do not know how we appear to others (we are all surprised when we hear or see ourselves on audiotape or videotape), it is probably more important for the ADD patient to see himself clearly. The Scottish poet Robert Burns observed in a very famous poem, "O wad some Pow'r the giftie gie us/To see oursels as ithers see us!," and continued in less well-known lines, "It wad frae monie a blunder free us,/An' foolish notion." The powers may have given us the opposite kind of gift: not to see ourselves as others see us. Many of us can get by without such self-observation, but the ADD adult cannot.

How education of the ADD adult is best accomplished and what kinds of therapy or therapies are best is not certain. Because our patients have had spouses or other partners, the approach we've used is derived from standard techniques of couple therapy. One examines the behavior of each partner, focusing especially on three aspects of the relationship: communication, expectations, and stylized patterns of behavior.

Frequently, marital partners have never learned to talk to each other—to say what they think, feel, and want. They hope that somehow their mates can read their minds. When this doesn't happen, they feel frustrated and become angry. Consequently, persuading marriage partners to say what is on their minds has been found therapeutically useful. Often just this step can result in some modification of behavior. Partners can also improve communication by making sure that when they do express themselves the other person has understood the message correctly—has the facts straight and understands the intention.

With better communication, the partners are also less likely to act in terms of unrealistic expectations derived from previous experiences in their own families or even from overromantic popular culture. Every member of a couple has to learn what the partner's actual desires and capabilities are, and sometimes this may mean modification of original rosy dreams about gourmet meals every day, athletic sexual performance on demand, and immaculate, well-behaved children.

In approaching established behavior patterns that may produce marital conflict, therapists help the partners explore such questions as who sets the household rules, whose friends are seen, who does what chores, who spends more time with the children, who decides how money is spent, and who initiates sexual activity. In examining important elements of their life together, the partners begin to recognize particular behaviors (from squeezing the toothpaste tube in the middle to overdrawing bank accounts) that have become sources of trouble. When the various irritants are brought into the open, the couple becomes aware of the need to compromise. Sometimes the therapist can help them by suggesting specific behavioral techniques, such as "bargaining contracts" or a "reward system," which can achieve a better division of household responsibilities.

When one member in a couple has ADD,RT, the kinds of problems that usually emerge in couple therapy are likely to be greater because of such factors as impulsivity and hot temper. The therapists's focus on better communication not only helps the couple to deal with the problems of living together but is an important part of the process whereby the ADD adult learns to identify individual difficulties.

Whether other techniques would be helpful needs to be determined. In particular, it might be very useful to treat ADD adults in groups. The group setting would provide the opportunity for them to observe their own and other ADD patients' behavior in the here and now—they and others can see the behavior as it happens. Group therapy can provide a variety of benefits: support and reassurance as the patients discover that their problems are not unique; an opportunity to express feelings that may be repressed at home or job, frank assessments of interpersonal behavior; a testing ground for experimenting with other ways of behaving, recognition and praise from others when behavioral improvement occurs; a situation in which the patient can be of help to others. In addition, when groups are composed of patients who are at various levels (from the novice to the patient who has already learned a great deal about his problems), valuable education can occur among the patients themelves.

Group techniques have been useful in teaching patients with various psychiatric disorders about their problems, the manifestation of these problems in everyday life, and their treatment. It is therefore very likely that group therapy would be helpful to ADD adults, but careful research is needed to demonstrate its usefulness.

Finally, it must be remembered that in addition to special difficulties associated with their disorder, ADD adults may have the kinds of other problems that anyone is likely to have. When ADD symptoms are controlled, some patients find themselves faced with problems that had remained hidden and that they now must tackle. However, a majority are pleased with the progress they have made and are content to face life's challenges with their newfound awareness of their specific problems and with their newfound help—medication.

7

Finding Help

As I have discussed, frequently problems that may be related to attention deficit disorder are first recognized in school by teachers, guidance counselors, or psychologists, who call the parents' attention to these problems. In some instances, the parents themselves begin to suspect that their child has behavior problems beyond the normal range. I wish to emphasize again that in either case, in order to ascertain the probable sources of the child's difficulties, the parents *must* consult a physician who is knowledgeable about the entire range of children's physical and emotional problems, including ADD.

If the parents do not already have a physician for the child and are wondering what kind of specialist to look for, they will find that the following kinds of physicians are most likely to be acquainted with the problems of ADD: child psychiatrists—M.D.s who have studied both adult and child psychiatry; child neurologists—M.D.s who have specialized in disorders of the nervous system in both adults and children; pediatricians—M.D.s who have specialized in diseases of children. Psychologists, who are not physicians, tend to be less familiar with the problems and cannot prescribe medication. The same comment holds true for social workers and school guidance counselors: they are helpful in dealing with any associated family problems that may be present, but they cannot offer medication, the most useful and sometimes the only treatment needed.

If the child's pediatrician is consulted, the parents should be aware that some pediatricians have little training in dealing with behavior problems. Parents should frankly ask the pediatrician if he or she does have familiarity with behavior problems and, if not, should ask for a recommendation to someone who might be more experienced in this field.

There is no foolproof way of finding a good physician, but several procedures may be helpful. If the parents live near a university medical school, they might first inquire if any of the senior staff see private patients. Physicians associated with medical schools are not necessarily better trained than physicians in the community. There are excellent, good, fair, poor, and incompetent doctors in both settings. The probability is greater, however, that a doctor chosen at random is well trained if he is associated with a medical school. Parents should first request that the child be seen by a child psychiatrist or child neurologist, or if these physicians are not available, by a psychiatrist who is familiar with the problems of children. If the physicians at the medical school do not see private patients, parents can inquire as to which physicians in the community had been chief residents in child psychiatry, psychiatry, or child neurology in years past. The chief resident, in general, is the trainee who has risen to the top of his group and has been considered qualified to assume, in effect, a junior staff position as chief of the other trainees.

If there is no university medical school available, parents should attempt to locate a directory of medical specialists that lists by state and city the kinds of physicians indicated above. Specialized diplomas and jobs, of course, do not guarantee excellence, but specialized training and experience in these areas increase the likelihood that the physician will be familiar with ADD and its treatment.

Parents can do several things to help the physician evaluate the child. The first is to obtain a written report from the school describing the child's behavior, his academic performance, and any psychological tests that may have been given. The next is to think about what the child's problems have been as he has developed from one stage to another, how they may have been associated with problems within the family, and what events or attitudes seem to have made them better or worse. Gathering information in this way will facilitate the physician's task.

After having discussed the problem with the physician, parents should feel free to inquire how much the consultation will cost and how many visits will be necessary.

Parents should also inquire whether the physician uses medication in the treatment of children. The question is necessary because not all child psychiatrists do use medication. Some avoid it as a matter of principle because they believe all behavior problems have psychological causation. Others, mainly adult psychiatrists, have not had experience in treating children with medication.

Inquiring of the physician how he or she treats children is sometimes difficult. Physicians tend (quite appropriately) to be somewhat suspicious about patients who question their manner of treatment. First, most physicians are beleaguered by patients who have read glowing reports of "Wondercillin" in popular magazines and come in requesting treatment that has often been undertested or overdramatized. Second, most physicians, understandably, do not feel that the patients should recommend the treatment. No physician in his or her right mind would remove a gallbladder simply because a patient requested it. This medical attitude carries over into psychiatry, even though it is the least scientific of the medical specialties and there is still considerable debate as to what treatment is best for what disorders. Finally, and perhaps most important, physicians have learned to be leery of patients who are "shopping around" for treatment. Physicians have learned from experience that many patients do not want to know the truth or the correct treatment and may try doctor after doctor until they find one who tells them what they want to hear. This happens in psychiatry and perhaps somewhat more often in child psychiatry. Some parents may want the doctor to tell them that the problem is only the child's problem. They may be unwilling to acknowledge that the relationship between themselves or between one of them and their child can affect the child's functioning. Such parents will search for a physician who agrees that the problem is totally within the child. Accordingly, many physicians have learned to suspect the parent who wants treatment only for the child. But the point here is that although almost all ADD children can benefit if the parents become aware of their own personal problems, this is not sufficient treatment for the ADD child. The parents must make certain that the physician is willing to examine problems that are within the child, that is, constitutional problems, as well as those between the child and the parents.

The parents must therefore in this case act in a way that is not customary in choosing a physician. In medicine, most well-trained physicians are in quite close agreement on how to treat most disorders. In psychiatry, since there is much less agreement and very little evidence concerning the effectiveness of various forms of treatment, any physician who claims certainty should be somewhat suspect. Some psychiatrists prefer medication, some individual psychotherapy, some group psychotherapy, some various combinations of these. There are many psychiatrists who are flexible and use different approaches with different patients or multiple approaches with the same patient. Other psychiatrists limit themselves to one approach or one sort of patient. Obviously, the chances of adequate treatment are better if a physician is not committed to only one approach. If the physician only gives medicine or never uses medicine, he or she is not the physician to choose. Thus, the parents should feel free to ask if the physician uses medicine in the treatment of children. If opposed in principle, the physician is not an open-minded student of child psychiatry. If the physician rarely uses medicine, or feels that it is rarely needed, he or she is probably committed to the school of thought that attributes most behavioral problems to psychological causes, and should not treat an ADD child. This kind of doctor would undoubtedly disagree vehemently with the recommendations in this book. I would argue that that physician has had relatively little experience in the use of medication with ADD children and is therefore not in an adequate position to judge its usefulness.

In any event the parents should remember certain principles that apply to any consultation with a physician. First, it is proper to inquire how long the treatment will last and how much it will cost. Second, it is always proper to request another consultation or evaluation. Third, if the treatment prescribed (medical or psychological) is not working at all after a reasonable period of time, say six months, another consultation should be requested. Fourth, it must be remembered that all problems are not solvable in all people, adults or children. Psychological techniques do not work in all people whose problems are psychological in origin, and medical treatments do not work in all people whose problems are physical in origin. However, parents should follow one of the oldest medical principles: if what is being done works, stick with it! If what is being done is not working, consider trying something else.

CUSTOMARY DIAGNOSTIC PROCEDURES

In order to give parents some feeling for what a good evaluation for ADD involves, I have listed below the diagnostic techniques usually employed. This summary is not meant to serve as a checklist but to convey to the parent some awareness of what adequate evaluation includes. I will also mention procedures that might be unnecessary or overly expensive in terms of the information they are likely to yield.

First, the physician will obtain a detailed history of the child, beginning with the mother's pregnancy and proceeding to the child's status at present. The purpose of the history is to determine the child's strengths and weaknesses, his assets and deficiencies, by finding out how he has gotten along with his parents, his siblings, his peers, and his teachers. Because parents often see different aspects of the child, physicians frequently try to have both parents present, at least during the early evaluations. Any other adults who have played a role in the child's upbringing—such as grandparents or full-time caretakers—are also generally asked to participate.

A very important aspect of the child's psychological history is his performance in school, both academically and socially. For this reason, most physicians like to obtain reports from the teacher (through rating scales, written descriptions, or conversation) describing the child's functioning in the classroom. This information is extremely valuable from several points of view. First, the teacher has seen many more children than the parents. Second, the teacher sees the child in comparison to his peers throughout his academic career. The teacher can determine if the child is advanced, behind, or at grade and age level with regard to both academic and social functioning. Third, the teacher observes the child's stressful developmental areas. The teacher knows if the child is having problems in learning, which can be a major area of difficulty for the child with ADD. Finally, the teacher observes the child's relationships with his peers, another frequent area of difficulty for the ADD child. Thus, the teacher's report gives the physician a much fuller picture of the child's functioning.

To expedite diagnosis, many physicians use standardized rating scales for both the parents and the teacher. Some physicians also use teacher and parent rating scales regularly throughout treatment in order to evaluate the child's progress.

Some physicians advise a neurological examination as a part of the diagnostic evaluation, but I want to emphasize that such an examination should not be done on a routine basis. Although physicians no longer believe, as they previously did, that ADD is the product of minimal brain damage, many educators still see the hyperactive or the learning disabled child as having neurological problems. As a result, they sometimes suggest a neurological examination. However, neurological examinations are now only performed when it is believed the child has a neurological disease (such as epilepsy) in addition to ADD. The child psychiatrist or pediatrician who is evaluating the ADD child will recommend such procedures only very infrequently. This avoids the need for expensive and unproductive neurological tests, including electroencephalograms and special X rays (such as the CAT scan). The electroencephalogram (EEG) has no routine diagnostic place in either the initial evaluation of a child with ADD or subsequent evaluations of changes that occur with treatment. Research is being done with specialized forms of EEG, but, if such procedures are suggested, the referring physician should clarify why they are being added to the routine examination of the child. In a clinical neurological examination, the physician seeks to assess the child's coordination and some aspects of his perception. If there is no question of *real* neurological disease, elaborate neurological tests merely quantify the nature of the coordination problems that can accompany ADD and do not add greatly to what can be learned by simpler methods.

Finally, any ADD child who is having academic difficulties—and perhaps *any* ADD child at least once—should be examined to determine whether or not specific developmental disorders (SDDs) of reading or arithmetic are present Such tests are usually performed by a psychologist and consist of two parts: an individually measured test of intelligence (an IQ test) and a test to measure performance. The scores on these two tests determine the presence or absence of specific developmental disorders. Although numerous other diagnostic tests are available to child psychologists, they are usually unnecessary for the evaluation of children with ADD.

The primary therapist of the child with ADD—the child psychiatrist—must often function not only as a therapist but as a coordinator, obtaining information about the child from various sources and prescribing several kinds of treatment—for example, drug treatment, parental counseling, educational evaluation (and perhaps special education), and sometimes psychotherapy for the child himself. Many child psychiatrists are trained to deliver and make referrals for this broad spectrum of services, but not all pediatricians have the background to do so. However, experienced pediatricians who treat ADD children recognize the need for these other types of treatment, and they too may work in direct consultation with psychologists, social workers, and educators trained in up-to-date treatment of ADD.

In sum, evaluation and treatment of the ADD child often require a combined therapeutic approach. It is imperative that the parents and all professionals involved in the care of the child understand the possible contributions of such diverse treatments as medication, behavioral techniques, counseling, and special education.

FINDING HELP FOR ADULT ATTENTION DEFICIT
DISORDER (ADD,RT)

Because the patient with adult ADD usually requires medication for satisfactory treatment, he must be treated by a physician. In addition, the physician must be able to distinguish between the symptoms of ADD,RT and similar symptoms seen in certain types of adult depression. The physicians who see most childhood ADD cases are obviously child psychiatrists, whose practice and experience with adult patients varies considerably. If the child psychiatrist works with few adult patients, he may feel uncomfortable with the necessary differential diagnosis. Adult psychiatrists may feel quite comfortable in the differential diagnosis of depression but not in the evaluation and treatment of ADD,RT, which has been identified only recently. What is needed is an adult psychiatrist who knows a reasonable amount about childhood disorders, or a child psychiatrist who knows a reasonable amount about diagnosis and treatment of adult patients. Other than that, no generalization can be made about which type of psychiatrist is best suited for treatment: it depends on the individual physician. Although family practitioners, internists, and neurologists can prescribe the necessary medication, they are usually not trained in nor comfortable in dealing with the problems of the ADD adult.

Psychological help for the ADD adult—like that for the child with ADD—is most effective when the patient's symptoms are controlled by medication. The physician who prescribes the medication may also be qualified to provide psychotherapy and may elect to supply it himself, or may recommend psychotherapy by another professional. Any such psychotherapist must have a good understanding of ADD in children and adults. Many psychotherapists have been taught that problems such as those seen with ADD are produced by psychological experience and can be corrected by psychological treatment alone. This is clearly not the case for both the ADD child and the ADD adult. What the therapist must focus on are the "bad" psychological habits the individual has developed in attempting to cope with his ADD. This way of looking at people's problems is comparatively new and not all accomplished psychotherapists are accustomed to working with patients in this way. Failure to be aware of the biological roots of these psychological problems—and the possibility of their relief by medication—can result in a faulty emphasis during psychotherapy. It is useless to examine the psychologial sources of biologically produced problems and to attempt to change them by psychological means alone. It is useful to help patients to identify their problems and any obstructive psychological habits that may be associated with their ADD,RT; in that way they can make use of appropriate psychological techniques in dealing with their troublesome symptoms.

As with the ADD child, it may be difficult to find a good therapist. The techniques suggested earlier in this chapter for finding an accomplished child therapist hold here as well—that is, inquiring at university medical schools or at local medical societies. The psychiatrists we have found most likely to be knowledgeable about adult ADD and its treatment have been those who have a biological approach and are particularly interested in disorders of mood, such as depression and mania. It is entirely legitimate to inquire of psychiatrists what their approach is and whether they consider themselves specialists (or semi-specialists) in the treatment of depression. Additional ways of obtaining an appropriate referral are to ask for one from the physician who is treating the ADD child, or to contact a clinic that specializes in the treatment of mood disorders. Until recently, such clinics have primarily been located in the departments of psychiatry of medical schools. Private clinics and specialists are beginning to appear, and some family physicians are able to make such referrals.

Help may also be obtained from nonprofit organizations interested in the diagnosis and treatment of related disorders. The Foundation for Depression and Manic-Depression is a nonprofit organization devoted to the education of the public about diagnosis and treatment of mood disorders; it supplies referrals to expert psychiatrists in different parts of the United States (7 East 67th Street, New York, N.Y. 10021; telephone: 212-772-3400). There is also the Association for Children and Adults with Learning Disabilities (4156 Library Road, Pittsburgh, PA 15234).

Shopping around may be necessary but it is useful. The ADD adult's symptoms may further diminish with age, but he may have them for a long time. An experienced physician can be an invaluable resource in helping the adult with ADD to function well and happily.

Index